THE FORBIDDEN ART OF SELF HEALING

THE FORBIDDEN ART OF SELF HEALING

Chet Anthony Johnson

ISBN 978-0-557-52863-9

Table of Contents

Disclaimer

By reading this book, you realize many things. The first thing you realize is that I am not a health care specialist, a doctor, a scientist, or anyone who has the qualifications to give medical advice; therefore, by reading this book, you realize that none of it the contents in this book are to be taken as advice. The information lain within this book is simply for entertainment value. This is for your leisure. I also state that there are no cures in this book, because the FDA has very strict guidelines as to what can be considered a cure. Only drugs can cure, and the FDA declares what is and what is not a drug. If you read the contents of this book, you must only do so with full agreement that all that you read is simply entertainment. You can even treat this information as opinionated. If you choose to engage in any of the practices mentioned in the book, you do so at your own risk, and Chet Anthony Johnson cannot be held liable for anything that may occur as a result of your engagement. By reading this book, you waive Chet Anthony Johnson from absolutely any liabilities or damages experienced as a result of having read this book or having been presented to it. Furthermore, absolutely no piece of this book may be copied, borrowed, stolen, or reproduced in any way without having received written consent by Chet Anthony Johnson. The only exception to this rule is in the case of reviews. If you wish to refer to parts of this book in a review, you may do so, but you must issue proper citation. © 2010, Chet Anthony Johnson.

I dedicate this to those who are passionate about healing, to those who dare to step outside of Plato's cave and experience sunlight for the first time, to those who dare to… dissent.

Introduction

We were born into bliss and thrust into the arms of a society that dared to keep us ignorant of our potential. You were taken from your healthy state of abundance and love, and you were taught many things which were not congruent to your nature. You were taught that the world is dangerous. You were taught that the majority is authority. You were taught to play by the rules. They wanted your innocence, your obedience, but they did not want you to think. They made you feel weak at school, they introduced you to diseases that never before existed and said that you were their receiver, they made your bed your best friend, and they prescribed pills to be your love affair.

It's the same story all over again. A baby is born into a healthy state of existence, it functions quite well in society, and it does not seem to display any limitations of ability; however, this child unfortunately grows up in a society that trains it to believe in reality and to never question it. This pattern of enslavement and break-away has been rampant throughout all of history.

Galileo was put under house arrest by the church for believing in Copernicus' findings about the sun being the center of our universe. Prometheus brought us fire, and he was persecuted for it. In the Christian religion, Jesus showed mankind the way to God, and he was sent to the cross. Time and time again, we hear about a society that is falling due to corruption. We hear about the mistruths, the cruelties, and the disgrace inflicted upon people by their rulers. There was a time when the tension would build up to such an extent that it would cause revolutions and revolts. The United States of America itself was formed as the result of a revolution against heavy taxation, serfdom, and dependency on an unruly king.

As time passed, leaders began to understand the psychology of human beings, and they realized that direct force would always cause revolts; therefore, the leaders became wise and they found wiser ways of controlling people by using subtle tactics. As a result, the television, news, misinformation taught in public schools, and a world that does not read have almost successfully turned humanity into a slave.

In this new kind of slavery, the victims are our minds. As long as they keep us strapped to our pills, our late night news of terrors, our knowledge of wars, as long as they keep us believing that there is absolutely nothing safe about the world, we will continue to die in masses. AIDS will find you, cancer will infect you, influenza will break you down, and lupus will deteriorate you. However, the story is not complete, because the universe exists in duality. There must be someone who brings back balance to all that is wrong, there has to be somebody who fixes the corruption, there has to be a dissenter.

I am that dissenter, and I am putting in your hands information that can save your life and the life of others. You will learn how to heal your body, you will learn how to get rid of diseases, you will learn how to take charge of your life, and you will learn how to break away from the chains and shackles they have locked you to.

I have to warn you now. The contents of this book will scar you for good, and if you do nothing but read from cover to cover, your entire vision of the world will completely be changed. Continue at your own risk. This journey is an all encompassing journey. You will learn the reasoning behind self healing, you will learn the concepts, the tactics, you will be guided toward your own path of health, and you will be taught how to take health into your own hands.

While you are traveling this route, I would like to advise you not to stop any medications you are currently on or to disregard a doctor's advice completely. Doctors are very, very, sincere people. They studied very hard in order to receive the knowledge they have. I truly believe doctors have your best interest in mind. You really have to take things realistically. The contents of this book will certainly bring you to such a level of health that you may never have to see a doctor again; however, please realize that it takes *time* to change a lifestyle. If you have a horrible tumor in your body, and your doctor tells you that it must be removed or else you will die, it would be VERY foolish of you to disregard that advice. If you need medical attention, go see your doctor. I do not like a lifestyle filled with medications, but if there is a certain medication that will save your life, you better take it. There is nonconformity, and then there is stupidity. Don't be a subscriber of the latter.

That having been said, I still want to offer to you my belief that the medical industry is a multibillion dollar industry. Doctors, pharmaceutical industries, and anybody working with health care is absolutely thinking about profit. Doctors have also been conditioned to think scientifically after years of training. They have been conditioned out of listening to their more intuitive faculties. Everything is considered in the terms of Newtonian physics of cause and effect. What I mean by this is that doctors have been taught to analyze situations on the surface level. They have been taught to treat symptoms instead of finding cures. There really is no profit in cures, so it's best to treat symptoms. In many cases, then, listening to your doctor could actually be detrimental for your health.

This book was written for you as an offering of hope. As much as I love doctors, I believe that there need to be changes made. I believe that we must adopt a deeper understanding of this universe. When a doctor pills you up, operates on you, gives you medicine to deal with the symptoms of other medications, and then tells you that you are going to die in six months anyway, you realize something catastrophic: you are not being treated on in order to be kept alive, you are being treated on in order to postpone death.

This book was written for the people who are told by their doctors that there is no hope for recovery, for those who live normal lives and simply want to avoid disease altogether, and for those with minor illnesses. Overall, this book is written for the fighter in you. If you are fighting a hard fight, and the world tells you can't do anything, I am going to tell you that the world is wrong. There is great power in your words, and I am going to make you a believer. You are going to realize how much power there is nestled within you.

Within these pages, you will find a way of life that will completely and utterly transform every single aspect of your being. Realize, however, that change takes *time*. This book is broken into many chapters, because it is very important that you completely focus all your energies into every chapter. Take this book as an instructive manual. Focus on each chapter, and try each concept before you move on. I would say that it is best for you to spend one day per chapter. In every chapter, there is a process for you to try. Complete that process. This book was written in such a way that you will virtually need to spend no money in order to get your life together. I do not like products that do not contain full answers. I do not like it when a product is made with the intention of promising you something great, but when you buy it, you realize that the product itself is just a sales promotion made for you to buy more products.

This book is an end unto itself. For the most part, everything in here can be performed without any extra money spent whatsoever;

therefore, there is absolutely no reason for you to not try each exercise as it comes across.

You will be taught concepts, methods, ways to apply those methods, and constant positive reinforcement. If you really want to read the book from cover to cover just to lull your curiosity, go for it. But, once you do that, please go back to the beginning and focus intently on every chapter until you have fully learned and applied its contents. My guarantee to you is that if you apply what is lain in this book, you will achieve massive heights of health you never before knew were possible.

If you constantly repeat the same things you've done all throughout your life, you will never get new results. It is time to try some new things. I believe that much of the information within this book will be new to you. Some of it may be heavy, and it may require a couple of readings. Just stay in there and really take in the information. It will be very beneficial to you.

Sincerely,
Chet Anthony Johnson

Religion and Faith

Note: This chapter may be skipped if you belong to no religion. I wrote this passage for those who are afraid about whether or not the teachings of this book will interfere with their religions. I am speaking from a Christian standpoint in this passage simply because this is my path in life. What I say here is not meant to change anyone's belief system. The teachings of this book are applicable to any religion without harming the beliefs of that religion. I can, however, only give Christian examples, because this is my belief system.

The concepts in this book are deep, scientific, and they are highly geared towards self healing. Because of the nature of this book, many of you might be thinking about impact it may make on one's religion. Will the teachings of this book interfere with your beliefs? Will they be against your religion? Well, let me first ask you how important life is to you. How important is your life? Are you willing to fight for it at all costs? This particular passage is really aimed at the people who are afraid that they may be sent to eternal damnation for learning such knowledge. If you are an atheist, you obviously do not need to read this chapter, so you may feel free to skip it. Like I said, this particular part is to take away the fears of those who belong to a religion. I speak out to Christians, Muslims, Buddhists, and all world religions. My examples will, however, be Christian because I can only speak from personal experience.

The Lordship of Jesus is a decision I personally made as a young adult, and I hold onto my convictions strongly. If you had shown me the principles in this book ten years ago, I would have pushed them aside because I want nothing to corrupt my vision of God. If you are wondering whether or not this book will go against your religion, just take my word for it. We have to realize that we live in amazing times right now. We live in a time when science and religion are colliding. As you will see in the principles lain within this book, religion and science mix very well together. I am writing about religion at the moment to teach you that you do not have to be afraid of learning this knowledge. As you will soon see, the teachings of the Bible are being confirmed my modern day physics, and your faith will be strengthened as a result of being exposed to this book. Forgive my ignorance, but I believe all world religions teach concepts similar to what we are about to learn here.

When you have faith, unwavering faith, your life will move in your favor. You need to keep fighting. Regardless of your views on religion, you have to have faith in yourself. Become absolutely responsible for your health. I have great peace of mind that I am protected by Jesus and my love for him. In the bible, it is written

> Your wound is incurable, your injury is beyond healing. There is no one to plead your cause, no remedy for your sore, no healing for you. All your allies have forgotten you; they care nothing for you. ... But I will restore you to health and heal your wounds. Jeremiah 30:12-14, 17

The funny thing is that there are concepts in Quantum Physics that teach the exact same belief systems! Continue on and learn how modern science is supporting your beliefs. Knowledge truly is power. I want to tell you to put your level of fight up, take my teachings, and then use what you learn in order to further accelerate your life.

When you stand up and fight, fight with your whole heart. Put your faith into everything that you do, and believe. When you speak to yourself, speak with full discipline, and demand that you expect the greatest out of yourself. Negative self talk will destroy you.

> Proverbs 18:21 "Death and Life are in the Power of the Tongue."

Through my studies of life and religion, I realized that there is absolute beauty in every single moment, that life truly is beautiful. I am reminded of the words of Albert Camus when he says, "in the depth of winter, I found there lay in me an invincible summer." There will be a moment when you wake up and find your invincible summer.

So, this is a call to your action! Have faith! Keep fighting for what you desire, and you will have it.

> 2 Corinthians 5:7 "We walk by faith not by sight."
> Romans 10:17 "The Just shall live by faith."

My father died of an unexpected heart attack at the young age of 44. A couple of months before that, my grandmother on my mother's side committed suicide. She had a life filled with agonizing pain due to years of sickness, surgeries, and arthritis. I've been through some pretty tough times in my life, yet my faith has always been strong. I am very strong, and I would love for you to not experience such outcomes. Life is beautiful, and you can live it beautifully if you try to.

My message to you is that you should never give up the fight. You should never quit. Your faith will take your strength to great heights. You have to have faith in what you are capable of achieving.

You mustn't ever give up the fight as long as there is a fight still left in you. When you have faith, you can move mountains. There is absolutely nothing that can stop you. Take, for instance, Lance Armstrong as an example. He fought testicular cancer TWICE, and he still won the Tour de France.

If you are ever in conflict with another person, try to solve the problem with love instead. In *How to Win Friends and Influence People*, Dale Carnegie fills chapters up talking about criticism. He teaches us that when we criticize others, we do not change their opinions. According to the laws of karma, what we do unto others is fired back at us. If you believe in science, you will realize that when you send out a vibration, that vibration must be matched as well. If you are a devout Christian, you know that we are taught to be kind our neighbors.

Do the techniques prescribed in this book, and just get over it. Life is beautiful. You live in wonderful times, and it is time to truly heal yourself. I learned some excellent techniques that I would love to share with you, and I also have proof about life after death. Do not be afraid as to whether or not this will interfere with your beliefs, because it won't. Keep reading, and you will learn how this book could possibly be the greatest book you could have ever read when it comes to strengthening your faith.

Chapter 1

Energy

The Hawaiians call it prana, the Japanese call it Ki, the Chinese call it Chi, and scientists call it energy. There is an interconnectedness amongst all things in existence. At the macroscopic level, there seems to be a detachment of various substances. For instance, we feel as though we are separate from the rest of the universe. A plane flying in the sky momentarily seems as though nothing can touch it, that it is truly free. Then we look at mountains that tower above grounds at staggering heights, we look at trees that cling to mud, we look at water that hugs ocean floors, and we say to ourselves that we truly are separate.

Looks, however, are absolutely deceiving. In the grand spectacle of observation, it would seem as though there is separateness in the universe; however, this is just an illusion we have convinced ourselves to accept. Western science has stopped at this illusory realm and dared not to travel further, because at the depth of existence there lies a staggering revelation which, if understood by the masses, could cause a transformational shift in the ripple of society's conscious infrastructure.

Billions, if not trillions, of dollars have been funneled into a system intentionally made to keep you dependent on drugs. In every civilization of the past, the breath of life was considered one of the most sacred areas of knowledge. Emperors of China held their breathing patterns so secret that a leak of information would result in the perpetrator to be sentenced to death. The reason for such procedures is that the quickest way to access this energy is through the breath.

Realize that every single substance in the universe is made of atoms. This has been proven time and time again; take a look at any modern day textbook, and you will see verification. All atoms consist of protons, neutrons, and electrons, all of which are different charges of energy; protons are positive charges, electrons are negative charges, and neutrons are neutrally charged. Most importantly, all these components are, themselves, different forms of energy. The smallest piece of existence to have ever been observed is the quark, which is nothing but a raw strand of energy.

Modern physics has made the concept of energy crazier than you could have ever imagined. You see, nobody has ever seen energy! Whenever somebody looks for energy, he or she only finds the forms of things energy becomes. It's process that never ends, it's the greatest chase. Scientists have been continuously trying to discover the root of existence, but they can never find it. The deeper they dig, the more distractions they see. One day, they may discover something a billion times smaller than the quark, and even then they will not have discovered the root of existence.

Furthermore, energy exists according to a rule called Werner Heisenberg's uncertainty principle . This principle states that it is impossible to determine a particle's position and momentum simultaneously. In essence, what this means is that you can see either where a particle ended up or where a particle is going. But, if you can see where a particle is going, you can never know where it will end up. If you try to see where a particle is at any exact position in time, you can never know how it got there. In Quantum Physics there are infinite possible ways for a particle to go from part A to part B. In a more fathomable example, imagine a baseball being thrown from the pitcher's mound to the batter. In normal circumstances, it would a straight toss. In Quantum Physics, however, the phenomenon is chaotic, because a game of baseball played at the quantum level would have an entirely different set of observations.

If a game of baseball were played at the quantum level, the observer could either see where the baseball would end up or the direction the baseball goes, but he or she could never ever notice both at the same time. For example, at the quantum level, a baseball thrown from the pitcher's mound could have travelled ten times around the world before reaching the batter's mound. Furthermore, **those who see the ball being thrown will absolutely never see the ball end up at the batter's mound. It won't go there. Instead, the ball will end up in one of the trillions of locations it could possible end up.** Where things get more chaotic and impressing is that **those who don't care about the process and simply imagine the ball being hit at the batter's mound will see the ball being struck 100% of the time, though they will never be able to know how it got there. PARTICLES CAN DISAPPEAR AND REAPPEAR FROM LOCATION TO LOCATION WITHOUT LEAVING A TRACE OF FOOTPRINTS!**

In Quantum Physics, such a phenomenon is known as the observer effect, and it is tied in with Heisenberg's uncertainty principle. To push the issue even further, we must understand another principle about energy, and this principle is known as Particle-Wave duality. For the longest time, there was a heated debate in science as to the form of energy. Scientists all over the world were beginning to realize that energy existed as particles and as waves. But, which form was correct? Did energy exist as particles, or did energy exist as waves? The answer was discovered at the turn of the century by scientists such as Einstein, Niels Bohr, Heisenberg, DeBroglie, and Schrodinger. The main prize goes to Schrodinger who came up with the wave equation, a concept too complicated to be discussed in the pages of this ebook.

Essentially, it was realized that energy can exist as **either** particles **or** as waves, but never both simultaneously. What's more astonishing is that the existence of energy dependent heavily on an observer. In other words, if you were to look into a field of energy and try to see particles, you would only see particles; however if you tried to see waves, you would see waves of endless possibility. And this here, my friend, is where all of the fun begins.

The main goal of this book is to teach you how to eradicate disease by focusing on the waves of possibility in this universe. Follow me, and let's learn the structures of belief, the duality of energy, and hands-on approaches that will take you to a state of health you never before knew was ever possible to attain.

Chapter 2

Yin and Yang

According to Chinese teachings, energy takes form in two variants which coexist all throughout the universe: yin and yang. The ancient Chinese gave the two energies opposing attributes. Yin is soft, Yang is hard. Yin is soul, Yang is body. Yin is life, Yang is embodiment. The list goes on. What's most important is to know where yin and yang are most influential. Yin exists in all that which cannot be seen. Your soul, your thoughts, your emotions, and your life are all yin. Ghosts and spirits fall into this category as well. Anything that appeals to the five senses, for the most part, contains yang energy. A rock, a scream, food, teeth, flesh, musical instruments, buildings, and water all have yang energy.

The combination of yin and yang is what brings forth life. All living things have yin and yang energies. You can imagine yin and yang to be similar to entwined black and white threads. These two forces immensely repel each other; therefore, when they are in proximity, there is a violent reaction which, if contained, springs forth life. When a baby is born, a violent reaction occurs in which the yang and yin forces wrap around each other so tightly that the black and white threads are indistinguishable from one another. The baby's skin is smooth and rich. As the baby grows up, its skin begins to slowly loosen. This is a sign of the threads unraveling. Once this baby reaches adulthood and old age, the threads are the loosest. Upon death, the threads are completely unraveled. The white thread, yin, is the soul and consciousness of the baby. The black thread is the body. The black thread stays behind while the white thread ascends.

This has been deemed to be the natural progression of life. We are born, we grow old, our skins sag, we lose our hair, our bones break, and we die; however, if we are to apply the laws of Quantum Physics as stated earlier, we do not have to fall victim to such an outcome. We realize that we are the creators of our realities, and that whatever we look for in the field of endless possibilities is exactly what we shall receive.

Further ahead in this book, you will learn techniques that will be used to strengthen the yin and yang entwinement so that you can age graciously, add at least another ten years to your life, and live with more vitality.

Chapter 3

The Conscious Body

Prevalent amongst all other forms of healing, conscious body practices are the strongest. The conscious body deals with the mind and the way it is used to observe the world around us. According to the Neruolinguistic Programming model of communication, the mind is exposed to over 2,000,000 bits of information per second. We are aware, however, of only, roughly, 11 main pieces of information: these include body heat, sense of balance, thoughts, feelings, the environment's temperature, and anything that appeals to the five senses. We really are massive filtration units. Furthermore, we are always choosing what information to let into our lives and what information to be blocked.

We are similar to radio receivers. Right now, absolutely every single channel in the world is playing in your room. If you get a strong enough radio, you can tune into absolutely any station. Your mind is the same way. If you were to tune into the frequency of your desire, that desire would be transmitted to you. Most people are consciously, and constantly, focusing on the very thing they do not want. When we think in terms of what we do not want, we create more of it. A perfect example to aide this scenario is me telling you not to think of a purple elephant. Of course, you just thought of a purple elephant. The mind cannot process a negative; therefore, any order the mind is constantly fed will be made manifest.

It was Carl Jung who said that "when an inner situation is not made conscious, it appears outside as fate." A thought harbored long enough in the banks of our conscious **will** manifest itself outwardly. Think back to the principles of quantum mechanics discussed earlier. Everything is made of energy; therefore, everything is subject to the laws and characteristics of energy. It just seems as though this is not the case because nobody sees instant changes on the macroscopic level. The truth, however, is that it takes much longer for you to see a change on the physical level if your belief isn't totally latched onto the manifestation. Everything has a gestation period. If a woman tries to get pregnant tonight, she should not expect the baby to appear for another 9 months. No amount of will power will bring the baby to fruition within the first trimester. It just won't work. Have patience, and allow things to manifest. More on manifestation will be discussed later. Just be aware about the role the mind plays on your reality.

In many ways, as you will learn soon, the diseases we have in our bodies are really inner situations not made conscious. Jealousy, rivalry, hatred, malice, guilt, sadness, depression, and helplessness can all, over time, transform into diseases. Realize, also, that disease means **dis-ease.** When a body has a disease, it is by definition out of harmony with all that is wonderful in the universe- i.e, the body is not at *ease*.

Jung also discovered what he came to label as the collective unconscious. He believed that everyone in the universe was connected to each other by this medium of consciousness in which thoughts flew in and out from all over and every which way. The ancients believed, like Jung, that everyone was connected. The principles of energy and Jung's discoveries have further accentuated the matter and verified what the ancients always believed: God and man are inseparable. We are all part of a great consciousness. Some call it God, some call it energy, and physicists call it the unified field. The unified field is, in essence, the root where all sciences collide. At the unified field, there is no distinction between you and I. We are all at our most enlightened state of blissful joy and oneness. The aim of enlightenment is to reach such a state.

Those who are diseased are far from experiencing Nirvana, but they can still certainly attain it in this lifetime if they were to take full control over their thoughts. In order to live this life to the fullest, one most learn how to take charge of his or her imaginative faculties. It truly means having a major conscious turn around.

Even in the physical body, there is evidence for such claims. The reticular activating system, the RAS, is a function in the brain responsible for taking orders from us and then working endlessly in order to find those patterns in the external world. One example would occur when you buy a new car and then somehow "magically" see that car everywhere on the highway.

If such an example is applied to disease, one can see why it may seem difficult to become healthy, because once you contract a disease you work endlessly to find that disease wherever you go. The truth of the matter is, every single possible reality we could ever live in surrounds us at every second of every day. We are like radio receivers, however, and we decide what channel to listen to. Most of us choose frequencies that weaken us. Do not be like them. Stand out from the crowd and choose not to conform.

You have the power to cure absolutely any disease, heal any relationship, and achieve any dream. There is absolutely nothing you cannot do. The higher ups in society do not want you to know about any of this, because it will turn you into someone who does not have to depend on the external world for sustenance any longer.

After this training, your world will become more like sandbox in which you may spend pleasurable amounts of time letting your life joyfully be lived in wonderful bursts of memories. Realize that your mind is everything, and it exists beyond your physical body. Who you truly are is magnificent, and you've been playing with weaker forces your whole life.

I like to use a concept I learned from James Arthur Ray in his Harmonic Wealth Home Study Course. According to concepts of electricity, power always flows from a higher source to a lower source. For example, if you plug in a 25 watt light bulb into your ceiling, you will get a 25 watt glow in the bulb. This 25 watts of energy does not represent all of the energy in the house. It's just the amount of energy you have allowed to be used in that particular spot. Energy ALWAYS flows from a higher source to a lower source. If you were to plug in a one thousand watt light bulb, you would get one thousand watts of energy in that particular spot, and that immense amount of energy still would not represent all of the energy that exists within the house. Even the water in your glass does not represent all of the water in your house. The container defines how much water can be received.

Consciousness comes from a source far greater than anything we can perceive, but most of all of humanity still focuses on perception. Most people look at the light bulb, and they think that this is all the light that will ever exist. And if that light goes out, they panic! They don't realize that a bigger light bulb could produce more light. They don't realize that a bigger glass of water could receive more water. They don't realize that by CHANGING THEIR THOUGHTS, THEY CHANGE REALITY.

Realize the greatness of your soul, and stop playing with illusions, because true power comes from within.

Chapter 4

The Law of Attraction

We must combine certain laws of the universe in order to explain a phenomenon known as the law of attraction. Subsequently, you will learn how to manifest whatever desire you wish to attain, most importantly, you will learn how to consciously eradicate disease by focusing more on health. The law of attraction states that whatever we hold in our feelings and thoughts constantly enough will manifest outwardly in reality. In order to prove such a notion, it is imperative that we focus on the laws of gravity, expectation, and existence.

Gravity exists in absolutely anything that has mass. Furthermore, the greater the mass of an object, the greater its field of gravity; therefore, Jupiter's gravitational orbit is far greater than that of Earth's, and both planets' gravitational orbits cower in comparison to the Sun's. Furthermore, even small pieces of matter have gravitational orbits and pulls. A piece of lint has a gravitational orbit, and so does a car. If you were to take these objects and place them in remote parts of the universe, you would find that particles smaller than the lint would orbit around it. You would also find small chunks of meteorites revolving around the car.

The reason why these phenomena do not occur on Earth, at least not on the macroscopic level, is that Earth's gravitational pull us so strong that instead of objects colliding and orbiting around each other, everything stays glued to the ground. There are, however, four forces in the universe, and gravity is one of the weakest forces. A force much stronger than gravity is electromagnetic force, and many scientists are beginning to believe that thoughts are made of this electromagnetic force. Gravity is unfathomably weaker than electromagnetic force. This is the first observation that thoughts affect waves of possibility.

Realize that you also have a gravitational orbit, because you also exhibit mass. Furthermore, we must also realize that absolutely everything in the universe is made of energy, as indicated earlier. The last thing you must do is place a test upon yourself. Think of your right knee cap without touching it. Eventually, you will start feeling sensations there. This goes to show that energy follows thought. Is it really that hard to believe? Your entire nervous system runs off of electricity, and it all originates in your brain.

If we are to combine these forces together, it goes to show us that energy follows thought, everything in the universe is made of energy, and absolutely everything has a gravitational pull. In essence, what this goes to show is that by thinking strong, consistent thoughts, we can change the gravitational forces of the universe and manifest desires in our favor.

Karl Pribram won the Nobel Prize for demonstrating that the mind is a holographic instrument and the universe is a construct of the mind. His theory is the Holonomic Theory which states that the world around is simply a system of representations interpreted by the mind and consciousness itself (Intuition.org).

The universe is certainly a series of collapsible and erectable waves that are contingent with our perceptions of reality. All in all, the combination of the previous forces goes on to demonstrate that our thoughts truly do affect reality. True power is bestowed upon the one who uses his or her thoughts for a specific purpose.

You've been using the law of attraction your whole life unconsciously, and you have been playing the victim role for most of this life. You've come to believe that you are destined for doom and that happy moments are only byproducts of luck. You have come to believe that life is a cruel place to live, and that there are many hardships; however life is meant to be joyous and abundant if you let it be. If you tune your receptors into the proper channels, you will realize a bliss you never knew could ever be attained. The key to all your riches, wellness, and happiness lies in your thoughts. You are going to be taught how to take this law of attraction and use it deliberately instead of unconsciously.

There certainly are many other ways of curing diseases, but the best way is always to come to terms with anything that is going on inside of your mind. The root of any disease is in your consciousness. Treating symptoms can cause temporary relief, but the problem is still there. You need to face that inner demon. If you combine the spiritual laws of life and use physical applications to further aide the process, theoretically, there should be no way any disease could ever exist within your body because a body that is at ease cannot, at the same time, be at dis-ease.

Chapter 5

Believing is Seeing

Quit trying to figure out the facts, quit trying to figure out how something will become accomplished. As I stated earlier, there are many laws that govern the universe. There are many principles that you must follow and be aware of; therefore it is vital that you understand! Life is meant to be a joy, it is meant to be blissful, and you must be operating from the greatest point of health possible to you. There are ZERO exceptions.

Earlier, I talked about energy and how it flows from higher sources to faculties. Most of the world operates from the lowest faculty of reason: perception. People believe their perceptions are reality, and, to an extent, they actually are. They are real because they make them real.

You must realize that your perceptions are only a small fraction of what reality could be like to you. You must learn to shift your focus and your attention to the very thing that you desire. There is a notion in the world that people use when it comes to factual information. They say, "I will believe it when I see it."

If we operate from such a standpoint, we will never achieve any great success in life. Look at some of the greatest people the world has ever known. If you examine their lives, you will realize that they operate from a completely different standpoint. They operate from the perspective of having a vision. They march down a road nobody has ever traveled, and they see what does not physically exist. To passersby, these people are blind because nobody can see the thing these individuals are following. The truth is, they are following a vision. The dream they have in their hearts is very real, and they are following that dream. They do not believe that things will change once they have enough evidence, because their vision is evidence is enough. You see, they operate from the standpoint of belief. They are the ones who say, "I will see it when I believe it." I like a quote I heard from

James Arthur Ray: "When the intention is clear, the manifestation will appear." When you operate from a psychology of belief, reality shifts.

When you truly believe in your vision, your wish must come true, because the mind cannot process a negative. This goes on to say that if you were to truly believe that you were absolutely healthy, then you would achieve health. Stop looking for the method as to how this can be achieved. If you reflect back on the uncertainty principle of energy, you will realize that the position and momentum of a particle cannot ever be simultaneously known. In the same sense, if you keep trying to figure out how your health will be made manifest, it will just prolong the process. By law of attraction, if you are constantly putting out a wave of uncertainty and doubt, doubt and uncertainty are what you will attract to your life.

You do not want this. You do not want to operate from a standpoint of disbelief and longing. Feel as though you have the very thing you are wishing for. If you do just this alone, if you truly believe that you are healthy, and if you keep up your positive attitude, providence will move in your favor, and you will not even need to read the rest of this book.

If you can take this lesson at its fullest value and truly take it in, then there is nothing else you will need to ever read again. You will never need another piece of medication. You will never need another pill. Your dream is real, and all dreams are real. When you put passion behind your dreams, it ignites them. Passion bursts your dreams into flames. You become like a flame in the darkness of the night, and all of your hopes and aspirations glow like beacons of hope.

Belief is powerful, and it is crucial for this game. We must change! We must change the way we think, the way we feel, the way we love, the way we carry ourselves. We must shut out the voices inside of our heads that are leading us to destruction. It is so important to operate from the heart, and to realize that you are the master of your fate is the greatest thing you could ever do for yourself.

Your dreams are valuable, and they will create the world around you. Your thoughts will filter your perception. What will you look for? In Neurolinguistic Programming, there is something known as the flashlight principle which basically states that if you are in a dark room in which there is evil on the left and good on the right, you have the opportunity to experience either. All you have to do is shine your flashlight to the side you wish to experience, and that will become your reality. You've been going through your life focusing on the wrong things.

Your focus has led you to where your state of body is today. Instead of focusing on your physicality, focus on your soul. Believe that you are healthy, and that is exactly what you will be. You will achieve such massive amounts of vitality that it will shock you.

Allow me to explain. You see, in the quantum universe, cause and effect happen simultaneously. In Newtonian physics, the world is a series of linear gestures. Everything seems to follow a straight, set, path. Quantum physics defies this, however. Quantum physics shows us, through mathematical insights, that time can flow backwards and forward. It shows us that cause and effect happen together. Furthermore, perception is induced by observation. In a field of particles, there are endless locations where any particular particle can be. Once you try to observe a particle, it must freeze in time. You always get what you look for.

The quantum world really is affected by our thoughts in more ways than you can imagine. Actually, it is affected by ALL the ways you can imagine! Believing truly is seeing. If you can believe it, there is absolutely no limit to what you can achieve. If there is one thing you take from this book, it is that you must always believe in yourself. You must believe in your vision, your dream, and your hopes and desires. Nobody else ever will.

Most people operate from their perceptions, and they believe that the thing they are witnessing is all that exists. It takes a very brave person to think otherwise. The perfect example is Plato's Allegory of the Cave. I will share with you this story in brief, because it really serves as an excellent example to drive my point home.

There is a cave in which people are chained to the floor. They have been sitting in this position their entire lives. They have never been able to turn around and look at what exists behind them, so they constantly stare at the wall in front of them. On the wall in front of them, there are many shadows. The people believe that these shadows represent all of reality, because this is all that they can see. Behind the people, there are huge torches. In front of the torches are the actual objects to which the shadows belong. The people have never seen these objects. Time passes, and one man gets curious. He begins to wonder if reality is all that he sees. He wonders if there is more to the world that is cast around him. All his life has started at shadows, and he had not known whether there was anything else out there.

One day, he manages to break out of the shackles, and the people get worried. They tell him the world is dangerous and that he must stay in the cave. The man says he must learn the truth. He turns around, and for the first time he sees fire. He sees it burning beautifully behind him on the torches. And, he witnesses the objects that are in front of those torches. For the first time, he realizes that what he saw before were just representations of what he is seeing now. He finally sees that the shadow belongs to something greater, something more concrete. He tries to teach this to his fellow people, but they do not listen. They do not want to learn new knowledge, because they are afraid. They want to cling to the comfort of their own safety, and risk means death to them.

The man decides that he is going to leave the cave to see what the world is like once and for all. They all try to stop him. They tell him that there is something known as a Sun which blinds people, and that he will die if he steps outside of this cave. He says he has to take the chance. He goes to the entrance of the cave, and there is a stairway going upwards. He climbs the stairway, and there is a boulder blocking his path. He pushes the boulder aside, and he sees a bright glow of light that burns his eyes, so he quickly pulls the boulder back and he goes back down to the cave.

The other cave dwellers accost him and tell him to not be so foolish again. They tell him to heed their warning and to stay just. The man does not listen. He goes back out toward the entrance, and he pushes the door aside. This is very easy for him now. He looks out, and he is once again blinded by the light. But, his eyes are most used to it now. He still shuts the door, and he walks away. The same scenario as before ensues.

He works the courage to go back to the door. This time, he sees the light, and he is able to accept it. He carries on, and he sees lush trees and grace. He sees a beautiful world and a beautiful blue sky. He is filled with joy, and he comes down to tell the fellow cave dwellers. They become very angry, because he is disturbing their peace. Other dwellers decide to join him. Eventually, the man is killed because he upset the system; however, knew knowledge was now learned.

That's the story in basic terms. And now, what I want you to know is that I've experienced a light as well. I've seen what humanity is capable of, and I want you to realize that you are capable of far more than you've given yourself credit for.

When you are using the law of attraction, you must fully believe that you have the very thing that you desire. Do not be fooled by the perception of reality, because reality is nothing but an illusion. Reality can be shifted by your thoughts. You have lived your whole life concentrating on the wrong things, and this has brought you much anguish and pain.

I must belabor the point and drive into your head that you are GREAT, and your dreams can be achieved. You must believe that you have the very thing that you desire. You must be like the man in that cave. You must realize that the world is fooled by shadows. You must be the one who breaks the shackles and sees the torches. You must see the objects the shadows belong to. And, when you are ready, you must push the boulder aside and see the sky.

In Plato's time, one could have been sentenced to death for having such knowledge. Plato, himself, was put to death because he rattled the cages of society. He upset the system. He would not stop questioning, and this caused major chaos in society. As long as people love their comforts and live in fear of change, they will always hate the dissenter.

However, you must dissent. You must strive for more than they are allowing you to. Scientifically, realize that your cells are dying and regenerating every single day. You lose billions of cells daily. Within 7 years, you are an entirely new person. Technically, the disease should have died along with the cells. But, your thoughts kept them around.

Believe that you are healthy, and it must be done. Really, believe in it. Make it a constant practice. The following passages will teach you how to keep up with that belief. You must constantly live in a field of excellence, and you must think in terms of what you WANT. Instead of thinking, "I don't want to be sick anymore", think "I have AMAZING health", because the mind cannot process a negative; therefore, if you state the former, you will inevitably get more and more sick. Speak in terms of what you desire. Oust the rest.

Chapter 6

Affirmations and Incantations

The first mode of attack we can use to get yourself back into excellence health is the usage of affirmations. You have probably heard this term being used thousands of times, because it is a word that is used by the self-help community in abundance. People are constantly referring to affirmations, but it seems as though nobody really knows how to use them. The term has become so jaded that it has almost lost its effect.

What exactly is an affirmation? What is the philosophy behind affirmations? Why use them? How do we use them? How can we most effectively use them TODAY in order to deliver the maximum impact? I, myself, disregarded affirmations for a very long time, because I thought they were weak. I did not think they could trigger any fathomable change in the fabric of reality, and that stating them would be a complete and utter waste of time.

An affirmation is basically a statement you recite to yourself at various times of the day in order to keep yourself on track. You have many affirmations already in your arsenal. Some of the affirmations you regularly use are, "I'm fat. I'm ugly. I'm sick. I am always going to be sick. Nobody likes me. I hate myself." It's amazing how well negative affirmations work, isn't it?

Well, the same goes for positive affirmations. The fact is, most people operate from the realm of victimhood. I absolutely love Neurolinguistic Programming (NLP), so I am going to introduce to you another principle from NLP called the cause-effect model. You see, most people live out their lives in the effect module. They believe everything *happens* to them. They believe they are victims to fate, and that their lives will inevitably end up wherever the wind blows. I would say that roughly 99% of the population is more or less this way. People really are big Debbie Downers. EVEN if you did not buy any of what I am saying in this book, even if you did not believe that negative thoughts have any baring on the body, wouldn't you agree that it's just more *fun* to live life with a positive attitude? The fact still remains, though, that your thoughts really do influence your reality.

You have been on unconscious autopilot most of your life, and your negative affirmations have caused you to become riddled with disease, poverty, and relationship problems. This is not good!

We must learn to take CHARGE of our minds. We must go on a complete rewiring process. You have to rewire your sets of beliefs, and you must condition yourself for absolute excellence. You really need to demand yourself back into health. You must have that soul and vigor to believe that you are already healthy. But, sometimes it is just hard to believe. Sometimes belief isn't enough. Sometimes we need an aide. This is where affirmations come in.

What you must do is pull out a 3 x 5 index card and a pen. Your affirmation must be stated in the present tense, and you must write from the viewpoint that you have already achieved the very thing you desire. You need to write down emotions, you need to state that you are happy and thankful. Then, you must carry this card everywhere you go. It is ABSOLUTELY essential that you read this card every single night right as you are falling asleep, and you must also read it the very thing in the morning. It is very important that you do it this way, because these times are when the unconscious mind is most susceptible to imprinting.

Remember, we are imprinting our minds here. It is an easy task, but you must be consistent. You have to do this every single day for 30 days before you can be totally rewired. It is ABSOLUTELY essential that you do this at least twice a day every day. If you skip one day, your brain will lose the pathways and you will need to start over the very next day as if it were day 1. It is very important, because it takes about 30 days for your mind to fully adjust to a new habit and make something into a constant ritual. You must make this a ritual for yourself. I am first going to give you an example of an affirmation, and then I will teach you how to write your own. Let's say you are inflicted with headaches on a daily basis and your name is Marie Gould.

On your 3 x 5 index card, you would write: "I, Marie Gould, am in a constant state of bliss, joy, ecstasy, and love. I am SO happy that I am enjoying the best health of my life, and I am very thankful for all the love that I constantly feel."

This affirmation is perfect! It shows states of emotions, it speaks from the present tense, it radiates passion, and it speaks from the tense that perfect health has already been achieved. The more this affirmation is recited, the stronger the affect will be. The fact, though, is that there must be energy during every single recitation. Inject your passion into it. Really feel the bliss. The universe MUST bend in your favor, then.

Now, it is time for you to write an affirmation of your own. Follow this template:

> "I, _name_, am so _state a positive feeling or emotion_ now that I am completely and abundantly healthy. I experience high levels of _state an emotion, a feeling, something extremely positive, etc_, and I am thankful for this."

You can write it in any way you like. You can add more emotion, you can add more positive words. Feel free to really spice this up. Do whatever I takes for you to feel as though you have experienced full health. DO NOT list the name of the disease in there. DO NOT say something like, "I am cured of _____", because your mind will be focused on that disease. Instead, just say that you are completely and perfectly healthy.

The next thing is, you must say this with PASSION. Tony Robbins dislikes using the word affirmations, because the term has become very jaded. He likes to use, what he calls, incantations. Incantations aren't magical spells. They are just affirmations BOOSTED with energy. When you state your affirmation, stand up and DEMAND yourself to be better. Shout it out at the top of your lungs. Hype yourself up. FEEL that energy. DEMAND of your subconscious that you feel better, that you are in the best state of energy of your life. Your passion will be so contagious that it will cause a quantum shift in your reality. If you can find no comfortable area to do this, do it when driving. While you are on the highway, SCREAM YOUR LUNGS out. When you are at home, say the affirmation with passion. If you can blast some music while saying it in order to drown your voice out while you shout, that is also acceptable. Make sure, though, that the music choice is right. Negative music also enacts on us like an affirmation, and it can be detrimental to us. Note: if you are in a place where you cannot scream, you may still whisper your affirmation and incantation. Just put the same amount of intention and attention behind it. Put the same amount of soul.

Whisper-scream, if you can. Realize that the FEELING is all that really matters. There is no point in screaming if there is no soul. Attitude is everything. If you can say something with true sincerity, if you can speak from your heart, then you can push the screaming aside. Just realize that you must do everything you can to make sure you **feel** your soul in what you say.

We must demand excellence out of ourselves. Why is it that we beat ourselves up when we do something bad, but we let our positive events slide by us almost unnoticed? Take CHARGE of your life. Take CHARGE of your destiny, and really feel the moment as if it has already been completed. Stand up, and FEEL that energy. FEEL that excitement.

Realize that the law of attraction is ALWAYS responding to feeling. You see, in universe, there is also another factor called resonance. Resonance is basically harmonization of energies. When different waves of energies collide into each other, if they are in each others' presence for a long enough time, they will eventually synchronize. This phenomenon of resonance occurs all throughout the universe. In a field of crickets, there will eventually be harmony. If you place a bunch of metronomes together that are beating in different rhythms, they will eventually match up.

When you FEEL good, you attract other good vibes to you. The universe matches out with that harmony, because absolutely everything must be in harmony. Whenever there is discord in your flow, the universe must deliver you more discord in order to balance you out; therefore it is absolutely essential that you feel amazing. You must feel positive as much as you can. It is not enough to simply say that you are positive. You must BELIEVE it. You must LIVE it. As NLP states, you MUST operate from a physiology and psychology of excellence. If you do this, providence will move in your favor, and doors where open up in places where you thought there was no entrance.

In order to achieve anything great in life, you must let go of your old ways of living and thinking. You must operate from excellence, and you must make your decisions be based on where you are GOING and now on where you have been. If you always do what you have always done, you will always get what you have always gotten. Take my advice and write out your affirmation/incantation. It will be one of the greatest things you could have ever done for yourself. When you recite these words, BELIEVE YOU ALREADY HAVE WHAT YOU DESIRE! DO NOT LOOK FOR HOW IT WILL MANIFEST. Remember Quantum Physics?

Also, realize something about the feeling you project with your body. When you are doing your affirmations, it is so important that you put yourself into the right attitude, that words don't even matter if the feeling is right.

According to the NLP model of communication, only seven percent of what you say comes out of your mouth. The other 93% is made up of body language and tonality. What this means it that WHAT you say is infinitesimal compared to HOW you say it and the way your body presents itself when the action is committed.

If are slouching, you have a big frown on your face, and you sound lethargic, what you say will have very little affect on your affirmation. When you affirm something, you are supposed to put your soul into it. Since the concept of affirmations is so jaded, Tony Robbins insists that you use incantations instead. When you perform your incantation, PUT YOUR WHOLE BODY into it. SCREAM it, POUND it into your essence. Demand of yourself excellence. DEMAND of yourself unwavering faith and persistence.

Stand with your back straight, your shoulders back, put a big smile on your face, look yourself in the mirror, and thrust energy into yourself. When you are driving, blast the music and scream your affirmations. Do you think I'm crazy? Well, you have been doing the wrong things your whole life. If you want to continue living at the level you are currently living, do nothing. Don't change. Don't do a damn thing.

If you truly want your health to improve, you are going to have to make changes. You are going to have to change the way you view the world, you are going to have to change the way you view yourself, and you are going to have to change the way you speak about yourself. You must set yourself up for so much success that it scares people.

You could scare disease away in this manner, because DIS-ease cannot function in a body that is AT ease. Once you put your whole soul into your healing, providence will move in your favor, and you will achieve levels of health you never before knew were possible. Pound your chest, walk with passion, and let your belief trample everything in your way. You defeat opposition by believing you have none.

Affirmations and incantations come in many forms. A personal one I would like to share comes from the bible itself in Peter 2:24: "Who Himself bore our sins in His own Body on the tree, that we, having died to sins, might live for righteousness-BY WHOSE STRIPES "YOU" WERE HEALED."

The word "were" is of course past-tense and indicates as far as God is concerned we are already healed...We have to be receivers its up to us to make this a reality in our bodies in our lives..

Now when it says "by whose stripes you were healed" it refers to the incident when the Romans took Jesus in Pilate's Judgment Hall and scourged Him with a leather whip. God at that time saw every disease of Mankind transferred (symbolically) to the body of Jesus through the lashes of the whip. Jesus was then taken to Calvary and was crucified. When they killed Him, they killed the sickness and disease. That is what is meant when it says "by whose stripes you were healed."

This is my primary focus point when ever I am in need of healing. I take ownership and make this personal, I state, I confess, I demand, I affirm what ever will make it plain to you but I constantly declare "By His Stripes "I am" Healed. This is done with much gratitude and praise and thanks to God.

Your incantation and affirmation work best when you have deep conviction in your heart that you are fully healed. The universe will work wonders for those who believe.

Chapter 7

Vision Boards

Let us REV UP the excellence. So far, you've learned a great deal of information. You really need to give yourself a pat on the back. I am so proud of you for having come this far. Have you written your affirmation yet? If not, GO BACK! WRITE IT. IT is so important that you Live your life based on WHERE YOU WANT TO GO. Start today. START NOW.

Are you done?

Okay, let's continue, then! I knew I could trust you.

So, we come to another piece of knowledge: vision boards. If you thought affirmation were nuts, you have no idea what you have gotten yourself into now. What are vision boards?! Vision boards are, in many ways, even stronger than affirmations. You see, the mind thinks in terms of pictures. Before language came about, man had to think in order to survive. Before words came about, he had to think in terms of images. In survival situations, words could not save the being, so he had to learn to think QUICKLY. Ideas came in the form of images, so he was able to make decisions quickly.

When you use affirmations, you are speaking to one of the most primitive parts of your brain. Really, your whole life is one big vision board. If I were to come to your house and take a look at your books, your posters, the movies in your collection, your music, and your collected goods, I would NEVER need to meet you to know what kind of person you are. Your world is constantly reflecting back to you the very thing which you are. If your world is chaotic, it means you are also chaotic.

We must do something to take care of this situation. We must speak to the most primitive part of our brains by using vision boards. A vision board is something you hang around your computer, your wall, your living room, or absolutely anywhere you spend your most time. Do not place it near a television set, because your mind will be focused more on the television that it will be on the board. You need to have a place where you can comfortably gaze at this board. It is best to have it nearby when you are falling asleep so that it is the last thing you see at night and the first thing you see when you wake up. On this vision board, you must put images of things that you desire. In this case, you must put down images of you in the perfect state of health. You must put down images of wellness, put down trees, put down love, put down happiness, put down joy. Put down images that bring you elation. Put up a picture of vigor, athleticism, people dancing, children jumping for you. You need to really put something fantastic up, something that really speaks to your heart and to your soul.

Take a moment out of every single day to just journey into the images of this vision board. Feel yourself there. What are the sounds? What are the sights? What can you smell? How does it feel to be absolutely in perfect health? Believe in your health. Focus on the very thing you desire.

The point of affirmations and vision boards is that you are finally beginning to live your life by conscious design. Living your life by design should be one of your biggest goals in life. You see, most people do not decide to take charge until they face a major dilemma. If you are severely sick, you start praying for health to such a degree that you actually experience it. Make it a law that you should always focus on, exactly, the thing which you desire.

The mind does not think in terms of negatives, because the mind cannot process a negative; therefore, do not give your mind commands of things you do not desire. Your mind is a genie, and it will process absolutely anything and everything you feed it. Most thoughts come and ago. The thoughts that are backed by the passionate fuel of your emotions are the ones you will see consistently manifest. What are you thinking?

This 30 day process of rewiring is something you must absolutely dedicate yourself to accomplishing. The vision boards and affirmations are quantum leaps towards the fulfillment of your health. Look at your vision board EVERY DAY, recite your incantation EVERY day. In psychology, there is something known as the law of five. If I want to know how much money you make and what state of health you are in, all I have to do is look at the salaries and health statuses of the five people you hang out with the most. You are the average of those five people. Your environment truly affects your body. It's not just people that affect us, but things affect us as well. Surround yourself with images of excellence.

Chapter 8

Intention and Attention

Energy flows where attention goes. When we discussed quantum physics earlier, we showed this to be true. We showed this to be a fact of the universe, and we learned much about the way energy works. There is still a LOT more left to be discussed, so hold on tightly because this ride is about to shift into a completely different stratosphere. You see, where you place your attention means more than you realize.

When you focus on something long enough, it causes that thing to expand. It causes that thing to grow. When you place intention behind it, providence moves the universe and places it at your footsteps. It is so important that you realize this that I had to make a passage for it in and of itself.

When you are doing your vision boards, when you are doing your affirmations, when you are doing your incantations, you MUST have SHARP intention and attention on what you desire. Sometimes, though these two tools are just not enough. A vision board isn't really an active element of your day, because all you do is look at you. The incantation is something very verbal, and it really requires a lot of energy.

There is a third way you can really unite your soul onto this path, and that is by obtaining a journal. You should grab a journal and label it "Why My Health Rocks", or you may write something similar to that. It is VERY important that you do NOT do this on the computer. Writing by hand is a much more active process than is typing on a keyboard. Many more muscles are involved when you use your hand. You really can feel your soul oozing out of your body when you put things on paper.

What I want you to do is write in this health journal from the perspective that you live the MOST vibrant, healthy, and joyful life in the universe. You must feel like you are a God amongst men. You must feel like Jesus, Buddha, Thoth, or anyone else you feel had stellar health. Hey, don't think Buddha was fat! He was actually in great shape. He is portrayed as fat because it is supposed to represent his abundance and joy. Buddha was actually a beautiful prince named Siddhartha, but I digress. Sometimes it's fun to digress, isn't it? I am experiencing tremendous joy writing this, and you should take in on the action. Have fun. Smile.

In this journal, write your life out the way it would be ideally. This is your dream book, but don't name it that! You want your unconscious mind to really understand that this is your reality. Give it a colorful name. You could name it, "My life's Journal". Your unconscious mind will absolutely believe that. Actually, your unconscious mind will believe anything you feed it. It's your CONSCIOUS mind that you have to convince. But, since your conscious mind is what'll be doing the convincing, this is going to be a very easy task for you.

Now, pick up your pencil and write! You have to become like a child once more. You have to get into that feeling of joy, ecstasy, and bliss. You have to live your life by design. I remember hearing somewhere that we have about 60,000 thoughts every single day, 95% of which are the same thoughts we think every other day. Imagine if you were to create new thought patterns every day! Imagine if you TRAINED yourself to spot out abundance and bliss and health. How much would your life transform?

Believing is seeing. Energy follows thought. Attention and intention mean everything. Where are you placing your focus? If you start writing these positivity journal entries, if you continue doing incantations and affirmations, if you jump into your vision board, your life will be stellar. You will have such a quantum leap in health that you won't know what hit you. Now, there is still definitely more to the story, so it is essential that you keep reading. If you do absolutely everything that is stated in this book, you will be experiencing quantum leaps in health. At first, it may seem like a lot of work, but STOP complaining. You've brought yourself here by thinking the wrong thoughts. Now, it's time to finally take control of your life once and for all. Isn't it time to break away from your strings, Pinnochio?

Okay, STOP! Go get that journal, and go make your vision board. No excuses. You made a promise that you would commit yourself to health. Well, go ahead and commit! If you really can't do it right now, then you may continue reading, but promise me, and promise yourself, that you will deliver. I can only show you the way. You are the one who must take action.

Chapter 9

Serenity

So, you have finally made it here, huh?! GOOD FOR YOU. What this means is that you have gotten your journal, you have made your affirmations and incantations, and you have gotten your vision board together! I really expect great things out of you, so if you haven't done these things yet, please go do them, because this next passage is about to get very practical; however, like I said before, if you really can't do these things right this second, feel free to read on, but promise yourself that you will get to them ASAP. Your health depends on it.

This passage deals with the passage of meditation. So, what exactly is meditation? Is it simply a pattern of breathing calmly in order to relax the mind? Is it a way to relax and focus the self? In a nutshell, it is all of these things, but there is certainly more to the story than they will let you in on. You see, as stated earlier, the Japanese call energy ki, the Chinese call it Chi, the Hawaiians call it Prana, and scientists call it Energy. More about these forces will be discussed later, but now would be a great time to step into the realm of energies as they deal with meditation.

When you meditate, you are becoming one with the universe. Your breath unites with the flow of the great force, and you become more and more centered until your soul beats with the heart of the Earth. At this level, you are immensely powerful. You will learn how to harness this energy in future passages. For now, it is good to have consciousness and awareness of the concept. When you meditate, your intention and attention are on your breath. Remember when I talked to you about the importance of breath earlier in the book? We are headed toward that. The breath, by many civilizations, has been considered sacred. I feel as though you are ready to step into a practical side of the conscious body's path to wholeness.

What we are going to be doing is digging into your soul and cutting away ties that no longer serve you. You see, one of the reasons disease is triggered, according to Huna beliefs, is by bad emotional garbage. Affirmations, vision boards, and journals help purify our thoughts; however, like Jung said earlier, when an internal conflict goes unresolved, it appears outside as fate. If you harbor any hatred toward any person, if there is buried guilt, if there is latent negativity towards another person nestled within you, it will certainly affect your health. In many cases, this negative relationship is the reason you aren't healthy in the first place.

Chapter 10

Introduction to Cause and Effect

I would like to share with you a very special meditation. I learned this information from Chris Howard's NLP Practitioner Training Series.

There are times when we feel lost, hopeless, stressed, and out of control. I am here to proclaim that every single person here is a God. We are all participators in this universe, and the life we live is completely under our control. For those of you who are burdened by the past, for those of you who are troubled by scholastic sorrows, for those of you who cannot move forward because there is a huge boulder tied to your back, this is for you.

You are extremely powerful, and there is a place deep within yourself where you realize this to be true; however, years of bad programming and conditioned insecurity have caused you to step away from who you truly are.

What is Huna?

Huna is Hawaiian spirituality. The ancients of Hawaii believed that every single thing in the universe is connected via an energy they declared to be known as akka. It is the energy that runs through our very souls, and it connects us to all that exists.

Wisps of threadlike energy connect us to every single object we touch, every single person we talk to, and every single experience we come across. The people, objects, and things we are closest to have the strongest wispy webs of energy connected to us, whereas irrelevant things barely have any discernible connection whatsoever; however, they are connected nonetheless.

Sexual encounters, obviously, rank in one of the highest strength bonds of akka, because during sex it is said that souls merge.

Using a special meditation, the ancients of Hawaii realized that they could literally take burdens away from their lives completely.

They could cause relationship wounds to completely heal. Ex lovers would be reunited. Ex friends would once again rejoice. Troubles of the past would disappear in the presence of this meditation. This meditation is known as The Forgiveness Process.

Uses:

1. Heal quarrels in a relationship with a lover, a friend, a family member. Used effectively, this can bring people together who have not spoken to each other in years.

2. Letting of of the grief of the dearly departed.

3. Eliminating stress, sadness, and pain, relinquishing any suffering we have within us so that we may once again feel powerful.

4. Letting go of someone we wish not to share our life experiences with anymore- be it a bully, an ex, a family member, etc.

5. Forgiveness of ourselves for past actions we cannot let go of because of the immense guilt.

You see, the huna believed that the world is a reflection of ourselves. They believed that problems begin within us, and that they are projected outside of us so that we may meet with them consciously. Some of the deepest, most profound esoteric huna texts would declare that we are the cause of absolutely every single thing that occurs in our life- the good, the bad, the ugly, the lovely.

YOU ARE THE CAUSE OF EVERY SINGLE THING THAT OCCURS IN YOUR LIFE

Now, I believe this to be 100 % true. I believe it, because it is empowering. It makes me responsible, and it gives me absolute control over my life.

There is a spectrum that looks like this:

Cause--Effect

Most people are on the effect side. They are always saying, "Why does so much bad stuff happen to me? Why can't I ever get a girlfriend? Why do I suck so much? Why does the worst stuff happen to me constantly? Why are bullies teasing me? Why am I constantly being laughed at? Why can't my boss pay me a higher salary?".

They choose to be on the effect side, and they limit their true potential. If we are to live in this life at all, why not live on the cause side of the equation. Those who live on the cause side of the equation speak in the manner of, "I am the reason for everything that is happening in my life. I take absolute responsibility for it. The reason I make 5 bucks is an hour is because I caused it to happen. I am the cause of me not having a girlfriend, and I will change it by doing missions every single day." Etc.

As long as we are human beings, we will always have problems. Who we choose to point the finger at...is another story. Blaming changes nothing. First of all, step to the cause side of the equation, and become absolutely responsible for all that occurs in your life. And if you are the cause, you can be the one who solves any dilemma.

You are the reason why you are rich, and you are the reason why you may one day go poor. The tide rises and falls constantly. We must never, ever, let our emotions be affected by it, however. True power is staying balanced even when the universe is storming around of us. We must stick fast to the center, and we must stay calm, and be the silent observer. While the mind travels a thousand words a minute, we must transcend the mind and simply....breathe. We must not let the negativity beseech us. We must not let doubt creep into our minds. And when we have wronged, we must forgive. And when we are wronged, we must forgive.

The Buddhists have a saying, which I am going to completely paraphrase:

> "Anger, frustration, sadness, sorrow, jealousy, and hatred are like hot coals- holding onto them will only cause us to be burned ourselves."

We must forgive others who have wronged us, because if we let ourselves become angry at their actions, it is a way of declaring that THEY have control over us. And by being angry, you automatically give that person control over your very mind, body, and soul.

Let it go.

We must constantly forgive. Forgive ourselves, forgive our lovers, forgive our enemies, forgive our friends. Forgive the world, and enter a state of love. You do not have to experience pain or sorrow. You do not have to let it get the best of you.

Let us begin, shall we?

Chapter 11

The Forgiveness Process

1. Find a quiet place where you will not be disturbed.

2. If you can find some calming, tranquil music, play it on loop. I love Pachelbel's canon. No lyrics, just meditative music. I love listening to canon, because it puts me into an altered state when I do this meditation. Just make sure it's on loop. If you can't find any music, silence is preferred.

3. Sit on the floor, or in a chair.

4. Relax your back, and close your eyes.

5. Breathe in and.....let the air fill your lungs.

6. Exhale.

7. Envision that you are outside under a bright, blue sky. You are standing on the ground.

8. Breathe.....In....Breathe out......

9. You start floating up to the sky. Really high!

10. Higher....

11. Higher...........

12. Are you breathing?

13. Go higher....

14. You are thousands of feet up in the sky, and you feel the wind blowing through your hair.

15. You look down and you construct a stage in your mind's eye. The stage is far below you..and it is huge.

16. A crowd of people forms in front of the stage. These are all the people you have ever met, and you are down there as well. These are all the people you share any sort of connection with, even if that connection is negative.

17. You feel the wind blowing, and you are breathing. You are smiling. You call up the first person to the stage.

18. You smile at that person, and you start breathing in green energy into your heart.

19. The person could be a friend, a lover, a bully, anyone. You look at that person and you say, "I forgive you. Do you forgive me?" Allow your heart center to spin clockwise.

20. If the person says no, say, "I'm sorry, please forgive me for creating this situation. Thank you, I love you." And then say to the person again, "I forgive you. Do you forgive me?". You should get a yes. If you do not, repeat this part of the process until you absolutely feel you have gotten a yes.

21. Smile, and call up the next person to the stage. Repeat the process.

22. Keep going until you have forgiven, and have been forgiven by, everyone. If it is a school, let that school stand on stage. This stage is huge, the school will fit. If it is an object, call it to stage.

23. Finally, call yourself up to the stage. You are floating thousands of feet up in the sky, and you look down and see yourself walking onto the stage. Thousands of feet up in the air, you look down and say to the You that is n the stage, "I forgive you, for everything. Do you forgive me?" Forgive yourself of all that you have hurt within yourself. Forgive yourself of past sorrows, past regrets, doubts, and insecurities. Forgive yourself, and reclaim your power to be a God amongst men.

24. Suddenly, all of the threads that connect you to all these people become visible. You see wispy web-like fibers connecting you to every single person on the stage.

25. A divine light comes in through your crown and it comes straight down into your body. You breathe it in, and your whole being fills up with love, forgiveness, and divinity. The light consists of the colors white, green, and yellow. And your entire being fills up

with them. Green is for love of the heart. Yellow is forgiveness, white is divinity.

26. The feeling becomes so great, the light is so powerful that it explodes and shoots out of your body and goes straight through the threadlike fibers and it flows down to the very people it connects to. You breathe in the light into every single person on stage.

27. Everybody fills up with love, forgiveness, and divinity.

28. And like a pendulum, two BIG blades come out of the sky, and they SWING from left to right in quick, sharp motions, severing all of the akka ties. All of the connections are severed, and the people fly off of the stage into the great universe ahead of them. The You that was on stage also flies away.

29. The divine light dissolves the stage and everything disappears into green love, yellow forgiveness, and white divinity.

30. You are in the sky, and the threads that were severed are still dangling from you. They are just limp and just waving in the wind.

31. You see a golden halo appear over your crown. It goes down....and it makes a buzzing sound. It is going down your head, then your neck, then it splits in two and goes down your shoulders, then it splits into five and goes aorund your fingers, then it turns back into two and goes up to your shoulders, and then it connects back at your neck and becomes one again. This halo is deleting the rest of the akka connections. It is purging all of the threadlike fibers. It is erasing them.

32. The halo goes down your torso, and it splits into two and goes down your legs. It goes down past your knees, purging along the way.

33. It splits into five for your toes, and then it comes back up to your legs as two entities.

34. The halo reverses the process, deleting every single thread by going upwards now. It does the shoulders, hands, then shoulders, and neck, and head again.

35. Once back up at your crown, the halo goes down and repeats the journey.

36. Do this once more. The halo has been done a total of three times now, and all of your akka are completely deleted.

37.   Breathe.....and let the love just explode inside of you.

38.   Start to descend from the sky.

39.   Count backwards from 10.

40.   Nine, you are falling.

41.   Eight, you are....falling, and you feel a part of you coming back to life.

42.   Seven, you are starting to experience subtleties in the five senses.

43.   Six, you begin to feel your body, and your consciousness is beginning to find its way to the surface.

44.   Five, you breathe, and you feel your body vibrating a feeling of love and prosperity.

45.   Four, your consciousness fills your entire being.

46.   Three, the green light, the white light, and the yellow light dance together inside of you like a flame. You feel what life truly feels like. You are on the ground now.

47.   Two, You are back in your body completely, and you are taking new...breaths.

48.   Open your eyes.

This meditation should take about 15 minutes to perform, and it is one of the most powerful ones I know. Try it, and you will be amazed at how you experience the world afterward. It should be performed once daily; however, if you cannot do this, definitely perform it when you feel as though you are losing control. We must constantly be forgiving. If you get emotional through this and start crying, keep crying! You are learning to let go of the negativity that has held you back for so long.

Performing this meditation really puts your soul at a sense of freedom. When we realize that we are 100% responsible for all that occurs in our reality, it gives us a sense of empowerment and inner peace. We finally feel the control we truly have. We become truly in charge of our fates. This meditation shines a light into our souls, and it cleanses us completely. It breaks away any bondage, and we feel the freedom of the universe light up within us. It is truly a blissful experience that you must experience to understand. If you do EVERYTHING in this chapter of consciousness- the vision boards, the affirmations, the journaling, and this 20 minute forgiveness process daily, your life will be COMPLETELY and UTTERLY revitalized. You will no longer be the same person anymore.

Sure, the setup may seem daunting, but once everything is situated, it only takes fifteen minutes out of your day to completely recite your incantation, jump into your vision board, and write a journal entry. You surely have enough time for a meditation, don't you?

Now, I realize you also have much other things to cater to in your life, so if you want me to ease up with the instruction, I will tell you that you can do away with having to do the forgiveness process daily; however, it is something you should DEFINITELY perform at least three times a week. It is important to break away from ties that no longer serve us. And, it is equally important for us to heal the ties that we wish could be better.

All healing starts from within. Once you perform the forgiveness process, you will finally begin to truly experience the divinity and purity that exists within your beautiful soul.

The conscious body is the most powerful, because it has access to the reservoirs of the universe. It is absolutely imperative that you take control of your thoughts and direct them towards more fulfilling routes. The next parts of the book will give you **very** important information as well, so really take all of it in.

In order to live your life at peak performances, it is really important for you to cater to all three organizations of life: The conscious body, the energy body, and the physical body. I believe this is also the order of their importance, because the physical body is just a vessel. I truly believe that consciousness exists forever, but that is a topic that goes beyond the scope of this book on health practices.

Chapter 12

Introduction to Chakras

Congratulations, because you have made it to a pivotal point of the book. If you thought things were crazy before, they are just about to get crazier. You are about to learn some very, very, deep esoteric stuff about how your body operates in the essence of this universe. Earlier, we talked about quantum mechanics, and the way the universe operates according to those principles, we talked about how energy follows thought, how attention and focus shape our realities, and much, much, more.

So far, we've only focused on the mind, and we have not really gone further than that. It is my belief that all problems and solutions exist simultaneously within the mind. But, since we are living a physical experience, it is still very, very, important to learn about what makes us who we are. You wanted a complete manual on health, so I am here to deliver. Now, realize that many of the concepts in this book ALONE can fill up thousands of pages. You do not need to learn absolutely all that excess knowledge. I will share with what you exactly what you need to know in order to achieve maximum health. I will also teach you things that will stretch your horizons and make you think of things in totally new ways.

Earlier in the book, I called myself the dissenter. I am going to pull you out of Plato's cave, so follow me as I show you sunlight for the first time. I am going to teach you about certain areas of your body that could crush mountains if you knew how to access them. These areas are known as Chakras, and if you keep reading, you will learn the what makes them important. So, let's take a deep breath and continue this journey.

Chakra is a Sanskrit word that literally translates to flat disc. Take a second and think of the weakest, most vital, parts of the human body. There is one area right at the center of the top of your skull, there is an area right between your eyebrows, there is the center of your throat, there is your solar plexus, there is your heart, there is your abdomen, and there is your anus. All of these are extremely vital organs. A strong enough blow to any of these can cause severe injury and even death. If you kick the anus hard enough, for instance, it can cause a heart attack because the two are connected. One shot to the neck, head, heart, abdomen, or solar plexus, and your life is most likely over.

Oddly enough, the universe loves to play a game of duality and opposites; therefore, in these areas of physically vital importance lie the strongest centers of the energy body. You see, there are seven main centers, Chakras, in your energy body. They are found where the weakest parts of the physical body exist. Interesting counterbalancing mechanism, right?

These chakras have special names. I will list you basic attributes of each for now, and then I will delve deeper into each one in the subsequent pages. Before we learn more about this, I would like to be clear that these chakras are only 7 out of possibly thousands. There are chakras, energy centers, all over your body. The practice of acupuncture serves as a way to accessing all of these energy centers. The pins and needles are placed in areas where there are meridians. Meridians are like blood veins, because energy runs through them. Since they are invisible, you it is essential that you get an acupuncturist or somebody who has the ability to sense fluctuations of energy to help you learn more about these. Like I said, we are going over the main points only, because these are the centers that matter the most. If you target these seven, not even death can take you.

Starting from the top:

7. The Crown Chakra: This is located at the top of your skull in the center where the skull is the weakest. Briefly stated, this chakra represents universal wisdom.

6. The Third Eye: This is located roughly a half inch above the bridge between your eyebrows. It is located right in the center of your forehead, and you can find it deep in this area inside of your brain just like the crown chakra. Hint: all chakras like to be inside of the body's central points in order to have harmony; therefore, you won't find them lingering on skin tissue. This chakra represents insight, telepathy, clairvoyance, the ability to see higher realms, and much more.

5. The Throat Chakra: This one is located in the center of your throat. It represents communication and being able to listen to your intuition.

4. The Heart Chakra: This one is located in the center of the body near the heart. This represents love, forgiveness, healing, and bliss. Many people neglect their heart chakras, and this results in a lot of disease. As a result, this book will focus heavily on the heart chakra, and this case was reflected in the huna meditation discussed earlier.

3. The Solar Plexus: This chakra deals with being in touch with the universe. It deals with letting go, it deals with manifesting will, and it deals with being in touch with your life's purpose. Tender focus will be applied here as well, because many people are also experiencing less than optimal levels of health because they feel as though they are victims to the universe.

2. The Dan Tien: The Dan Tien is located in the abdomen. The abdomen is three inches below the naval and three inches inward. This is the elixir field of the body. The ancients believed this to be the most important chakra, and they said that the center of the universe lies in this spot. This is an extremely important chakra to discuss, so be prepared to have a huge lesson hammered into you soon. You are going to learn about ghosts, celestial entities, immortality,

1. The Root Chakra: This is found around your anus, and it connects you to the Earth. It lets you feel connected to all that is around you, and it allows you to flow with the rhythm of the universe.

All of the chakras have special colors as well, and we will get into all of the fun stuff momentarily. Realize for now that these seven are what you will absolutely need to work with if you want to get into the greatest health of your life. This book is taking a different direction now. You see, at this level, not only will you achieve well being, but you will also super charge your very essence. You are stepping into a completely different realm now.

Chapter 13

The Crown

The Crown chakra is located at the top of the head, as stated before. Its color is violet. So far, we've been pretty much concerned with the crown chakra, but we still have not dealt with it directly. This chakra is a flat disc that spins clockwise. Its function is universal intelligence. When somebody's crown chakra is in balance, he or she receives flashes of insight from time to time. When people have super charged crown chakras, however, they can be seen as geniuses.

Everybody is born with certain chakras more awake then the others. Somebody who was born was a very powerful crown chakra can, by all intents and purposes, be considered to be a genius. This person has access to universal knowledge. Information just comes to him or her with ease. People who have this chakra awakened to a powerful extent feel the rhythm of the universe. They feel at ease, and they know that everything is working perfectly. And, what else could be better? The ancients said that those who have an awakened crown chakra can experience God. If you are an atheist, you will experience a more awakened sense of being. Matter of fact, this is an understatement, because you will feel the oneness of the universe. You will feel connected to absolutely everything that exists, and that is absolutely one of the greatest feelings you could achieve.

The people whose crown chakras are COMPLETELY awake can reach the highest states of enlightenment, and they reach a state of existence where the higher planes and physical planes (more on this later) mesh. I would like to think that Matt Damon's crown chakra was quite supercharged in Good Will Hunting. When the crown chakra is out of order, there can be paranoia, headaches, confusion, mental irritation, and disconnectedness from the universe. I will now provide a meditation for this chakra which can be performed in order to awaken it. This meditation is very powerful, but it takes time to get used to. At first, you might just feel pins and needles, but if you continue practicing, you will experience heavy, heavy, evolution in your mental faculties. It is essential that you find a place to meditate daily. You need to find a place where you do nothing but meditate. If this place happens to be your bedroom, so be it. Just designate a particular spot of your bedroom to be your meditation spot. Keep this area very clean. *Don't* meditate on your bed, because you have conditioned yourself to fall asleep in bed.

The Crown Chakra Meditation

Wear loose, comfortable clothing. Put up a *Do Not Disturb* sign on your door, or let people know that you need your peace and that you must be left alone for at least 20 minutes.

1.   Close your eyes, and take in a deep breath while slowly counting to four.

2.   Exhale for a count of four, rest your arms on your lap, cross your legs, and hold your hands in such a way that your right fingers rest on your left fingers, and your thumbs rest on top of each other, creating a big circle. Let this rest in front of your abdomen.

3.   Place the tip of your tongue to the roof of your mouth, and keep it as such for the duration of the exercise. Keep your mouth closed, and only breathe through your nose.

4.   Repeat this breath cycle as such for 30 cycles. What this will do is get your mind and body into synchronization. This is absolutely important, because this is one of the beginning stages of feeling the oneness of the universe.

5.   Breathe in, and visualize a flat, violet, disc in the middle of your crown. The flat side of this disc is facing forward instead of facing the ceiling. Visualize, and feel, violet orbs of energy going through your nostrils and flowing straight into your crown chakra. As you are inhaling, also allow violet energy from the universe to vortex into the crown chakra directly through your crown.

6.   Let the energy gather there. When you exhale, visualize, and FEEL, that the crown chakra is spinning clockwise. It is spinning slowly.

7. Repeat steps five and six for the next 20 minutes, but let the chakra spin faster upon every exhale. Make sure the inhales and exhales are both the same duration and length as they were at the beginning of the exercise.

Chapter 14

The Third Eye

The Third Eye is a very interesting chakra. This is the chakra that allows you to see into higher realms (like I said, these will be explained later). The third eye chakra allows you to see auras. Energy fields are finally open to you. You will see things your physical two eyes could never see. You can see peoples' intentions. You can see where a person's energy is headed. If somebody is about to attack another person, you can see the intention of that person's energy flowing toward the target. You have a finer intuition about things in life, and you can see the interconnectedness of the universe.

The Third Eye is truly a psychic chakra. Your psychic abilities are unleashed profoundly through the usage of this chakra. You have a greater understanding of yourself, and you feel powerful. You have more clarity over your thoughts, and you get to experience higher realms of functioning. Your dreams are more clear, and you have greater ease in having out of body experiences.

Because of the power of this chakra, there are also severe problems that can occur if it is out of balance. You can experience fevers, infections, irritability in mood, your intuition plummets, and you begin making horrible decisions in life. You are completely out of alignment with the universe and the higher forces that operate within you. It is imperative that you get this chakra in order.

You need to have that kind of control in your life. Those who have evolved third eye chakras can read the patterns of energy. They can see where it is headed. Since everything in the universe is vibration and energy, people who have evolved third eye chakras can also go ahead and predict the future quiet accurately. It takes practice, but it is definitely a pursuit that is worth it.

The third eye chakra is a royal blue color, and it is located in the center of the head, and it is right behind the center of the forehead. This chakra also spins clockwise. The meditation for it almost exactly the same as the other chakra meditations. Since this book is meant to be taken as a reference manual as well as an informative text, I will reproduce the slightly varied meditations for all chakras as they come by.

The Third Eye Meditation

1. Close your eyes, and take in a deep breath while slowly counting to four.

2. Exhale for a count of four, rest your arms on your lap, cross your legs, and hold your hands in such a way that your right fingers rest on your left fingers, and your thumbs rest on top of each other, creating a big circle. Let this rest in front of your abdomen.

3. Place the tip of your tongue to the roof of your mouth, and keep it as such for the duration of the exercise. Keep your mouth closed, and only breathe through your nose.

4. Repeat this breath cycle as such for 30 cycles. What this will do is get your mind and body into synchronization. This is absolutely important, because this is one of the beginning stages of feeling the oneness of the universe.

5. Breathe in, and visualize a flat, royal blue, disc in the middle of your forehead. The flat side of this disc is facing forward instead of facing the ceiling. Visualize, and feel, royal blue orbs of energy going through your nostrils and flowing straight into your third eye chakra. As you are inhaling, also allow royal blue energy from the universe to vortex into the third eye chakra directly through your third eye.

6. Let the energy gather there. When you exhale, visualize, and FEEL, that the third eye chakra is spinning clockwise. It is spinning slowly.

7. Repeat steps five and six for the next 20 minutes, but let the chakra spin faster upon every exhale. Make sure the inhales and exhales are both the same duration and length as they were at the beginning of the exercise.

Chapter 15

The Throat

The throat chakra is a rather fascinating chakra as well. This happens to deal with focusing on your inner voice and being able to trust it. This is the place where intuition actually speaks to you. You have to be able to listen to it, though. You have to be able to hear it out. You have to be able to trust it.

When you are taking a test, there are times when you get a slight hunch of what the answer could be. This is usually your first guess. If you strengthen your throat chakra, it will allow you to listen to that inner voice more sharply.

The throat chakra also allows you to express yourself more fully. When this chakra is awake, you speak with more clarity, people understand you better, you have more confidence behind your voice. You are able to put together words more efficiently, you are truly able to *flow*. Passion excites out of you. If you are writing a song, the right lyrics come out of you. If you are delivering a speech, the right words form. It's almost instantaneous, and it's quite freaky.

When dealing with sickness, the throat chakra will allow you to follow your intuition more closely. It will direct you to the right people, it will give you sources of inspiration, and it will allow you to know and feel that absolutely everything is alright. You feel the inner communication and guidance evolve, and you truly feel nurtured.

When you are taking tests, you will more easily answer questions. You will have a stronger gut instinct as to what an answer might be if you do not consciously know it. This helps you to study for exams much better, and it makes your health improve dramatically because you are listening to a higher, more positive part of yourself. Negative self talk seems to die when in presence of the love of an evolved throat chakra.

The color of this chakra is ice blue, and it is located in the center of the throat. It is also a flat disc that spins clockwise.

The Throat Chakra Meditation

The heart chakra is located in the center of the chest, above the solar plexus, below the throat. It is a pale green chakra, and it is supposed to represent love. The meditation is exactly the same as the meditation for the other chakras, but this time, you focus on the heart instead. Instead of focusing on violet energy, you focus on pale green energy.

1.   Close your eyes, and take in a deep breath while slowly counting to four.

2.   Exhale for a count of four, rest your arms on your lap, cross your legs, and hold your hands in such a way that your right fingers rest on your left fingers, and your thumbs rest on top of each other, creating a big circle. Let this rest in front of your abdomen.

3.   Place the tip of your tongue to the roof of your mouth, and keep it as such for the duration of the exercise. Keep your mouth closed, and only breathe through your nose.

4.   Repeat this breath cycle as such for 30 cycles. What this will do is get your mind and body into synchronization. This is absolutely important, because this is one of the beginning stages of feeling the oneness of the universe.

5.   Breathe in, and visualize a flat, ice blue, disc in the middle of your throat. The flat side of this disc is facing forward instead of facing the ceiling. Visualize, and feel, ice blue orbs of energy going through your nostrils and flowing straight into your throat chakra. As you are inhaling, also allow ice blue energy from the universe to vortex into the throat chakra directly through your throat.

6.   Let the energy gather there. When you exhale, visualize, and FEEL, that the throat chakra is spinning clockwise. It is spinning slowly.

7.   Repeat steps five and six for the next 20 minutes, but let the chakra spin faster upon every exhale. Make sure the inhales and exhales are both the same duration and length as they were at the beginning of the exercise.

Chapter 16

The Heart

The heart chakra deals with love and passion. When you have the heart chakra in balance, you will feel as though there is only peace in the world. When you are around others, their souls will light up in your presence. You will stimulate the environment by your message of inner peace. You will not even have to speak a word, and people will feel your love. The forgiveness process shared earlier was aimed at the heart. When you have compassion and love, all hatred dies.

There is something known as the Maharishi Effect. It was discovered that when a group of people meditates in unison, the affect is felt all over the world. Your vibes send out into the universe, and other vibrations must match the love you are sending out. More on this will be explained later; just realize that your energy is felt all over.

When your heart is energized, malice goes away. Feelings of guilt die, and you are truly joyful. When you are in a state of true, divine, love, disease cannot touch you. This is especially amazing. Relationships heal automatically. Those that do not serve you dissipate. The forgiveness process was more of an external method, because you focused on things outside of you for healing. The meditation we are about to experience now will be aimed at the heart entirely.

When you meditate with the heart, you can feel your passion bubbling out of you, and at very high levels of this, you feel unbelievably joyful. When your heart chakra is out of balance, you experience much negativity. You experience hatred for the world. You also have problems such as heart attacks, lack of desire, lifelessness, lack of passion, and stress boils up.

I believe that almost all disease is triggered by stress, and stress causes our bodies to fall out of ease; therefore it is essential to have a fully awakened heart chakra. At the highest levels of heart awakening, you experience such love and beauty in the world that your life is completely transformed. You could walk outside in a field, and exotic animals will want your company. Mother nature will not fear you because fear does not exist within your heart.

The Heart Chakra Meditation

The heart chakra is located in the center of the chest, above the solar plexus, below the throat. It is a pale green chakra, and it is supposed to represent love. The meditation is exactly the same as the meditation for the other chakras, but this time, you focus on the heart instead. Instead of focusing on violet energy, you focus on pale green energy.

1. Close your eyes, and take in a deep breath while slowly counting to four.

2. Exhale for a count of four, rest your arms on your lap, cross your legs, and hold your hands in such a way that your right fingers rest on your left fingers, and your thumbs rest on top of each other, creating a big circle. Let this rest in front of your abdomen.

3. Place the tip of your tongue to the roof of your mouth, and keep it as such for the duration of the exercise. Keep your mouth closed, and only breathe through your nose.

4. Repeat this breath cycle as such for 30 cycles. What this will do is get your mind and body into synchronization. This is absolutely important, because this is one of the beginning stages of feeling the oneness of the universe.

5. Breathe in, and visualize a flat, pale green, disc in the middle of your chest. The flat side of this disc is facing forward instead of facing the ceiling. Visualize, and feel, pale green orbs of energy going through your nostrils and flowing straight into your heart chakra. As you are inhaling, also allow pale green energy from the universe to vortex into the heart chakra directly through your heart.

6. Let the energy gather there. When you exhale, visualize, and FEEL, that the heart chakra is spinning clockwise. It is spinning slowly.

7. Repeat steps five and six for the next 20 minutes, but let the chakra spin faster upon every exhale. Make sure the inhales and exhales are both the same duration and length as they were at the beginning of the exercise.

Chapter 17

The Solar Plexus

One of the biggest reasons you are not in optimum health could be that your solar plexus chakra is not in harmony. This may be one of the most important chakras for you to take into consideration. You see, when your solar plexus is out of alignment, you yourself feel as though you have no control over absolutely anything in your life. You feel as though life is a series of events which you are a victim to.

We spoke about the law of attraction earlier. We talked about how you can manifest absolutely any desire you wish, and that you must be steadfast on the feeling that you have already attained that which you desire. The solar plexus chakra can increase this feeling exponentially.

This chakra deals with manifestation of will. At the highest levels of its awakening, you experience that you are a soul having a physical experience, and that the body is just your vessel. You really feel at complete control over everything, because you realize that the world I just a reflection of your inner states anyway.

Whatever you desire will manifest. If you were to JUST meditate on this chakra alone, it would give you profound changes to your health. The changes will be so amazing that you won't even know what hit you. Actually, you *will* know, because you willed it to happen!

When this chakra is out of balance, you can have diabetes, blood problems, and tons of unfortunate events. You will see the world as a cruel place, and the worst part is that you won't even know that you are causing all of it to happen. Fix this chakra, and you will take a quantum leap towards having the best health imaginable.

The solar plexus chakra is located right below your sternum. At the bottom of your sternum, there is a small hole. It's big enough for your index finger to perfectly match. If you push in, you will feel the point. A few inches inwardly, you will find your Solar Plexus Chakra.

The Solar Plexus Chakra Meditation

The Solar Plexus is a pale yellow chakra; therefore, when you are meditating, visualize all the important components to be pale yellow.

1. Close your eyes, and take in a deep breath while slowly counting to four.

2. Exhale for a count of four, rest your arms on your lap, cross your legs, and hold your hands in such a way that your right fingers rest on your left fingers, and your thumbs rest on top of each other, creating a big circle. Let this rest in front of your abdomen.

3. Place the tip of your tongue to the roof of your mouth, and keep it as such for the duration of the exercise. Keep your mouth closed, and only breathe through your nose.

4. Repeat this breath cycle as such for 30 cycles. What this will do is get your mind and body into synchronization. This is absolutely important, because this is one of the beginning stages of feeling the oneness of the universe.

5. Breathe in, and visualize a flat, pale yellow, disc right below your sternum, behind your solar plexus. The flat side of this disc is facing forward instead of facing the ceiling. Visualize, and feel, pale yellow orbs of energy going through your nostrils and flowing straight into your solar plexus chakra. As you are inhaling, also allow pale yellow energy from the universe to vortex into the solar plexus chakra directly through your solar plexus.

6. Let the energy gather there. When you exhale, visualize, and FEEL, that the solar plexus chakra is spinning clockwise. It is spinning slowly.

7. Repeat steps five and six for the next 20 minutes, but let the chakra spin faster upon every exhale. Make sure the inhales and exhales are both the same duration and length as they were at the beginning of the exercise.

Chapter 18

The Dan Tien

The dan tien has been considered to be one of the most sacred chakras in the spiritual body. The Chinese believed it to be the center of the universe. This is truly the center of the spiritual body. This chakra connects you to the greatest power within your soul. This is where energies harmonize. This is where birth and reproduction come from.

Yin and yang unite in the dan tien. Yin is very cold, and yang is very hot. The dan tien, itself, is yang energy. When enough energy is stored in the dan tien, you can feel your body begin to burn. It almost feels like fire. It's a fire that does not burn. The field that directly surrounds the dan tien, as taught by Kosta Danoas in *The Magus of Java*, is purely yin. This is how the dan tien stays in place.

When your dan tien is strong enough, you can tap objects and cause them to disintegrate. Great sexual energy is harnessed in the dan tien. If you go for a while without engaging in any sexual activity or sexual fluid release, you can feel the heat of this chakra automatically build up. This energy stays deposited in the dan tien, and it continues to grow. The yang energy gets hotter and hotter, and it wants to find a way to neutralize. The quickest way for this energy to neutralize is by leaving your body into the yin of the universe; therefore, sexual desire skyrockets.

Pay VERY close attention, because your life really depends on it. You see, your solar plexus chakra deals with sexual desire. Your sexual energy is one of the strongest forces in your system. You can see the power of sexual energy when you neuter a dangerous dog, because it becomes completely docile. Sexual energy causes us to do great things. No, let me restate that. Sexual energy CAN cause us to do great things.

Most people waste it, though. They let the sexual energy seep out of them, and they feel drained. Men who practice masturbation are the greatest victims to this. Realize that one amount of ejaculation has enough sperm to produce over 300 million babies. That's the entire population of the United States. Men have THIS much power within them, and most of them waste it. It really puts a great toll on your body when you lose this energy. The essence of your sperm comes from your heart, your liver, your brain, and other precious organs. When this reserve is depleted, your whole body is taxed and more energy is taken from it. Loss of sexual energy causes you to age faster, it can cause disease to be born, and it really depletes your very essence.

Therefore, it is essential that you learn sacred sexual techniques in order to slow down this release. The best thing you can do is realize that energy flows where attention goes. If you must engage in sexual activity, imagine that the fluid is going up through your spine as opposed to out of your body. This will redirect the yang energy and take it to a more invigorating route.

The sexual energy is very powerful. If you can learn to use it for purposes other than sexual purposes, you can conquer nations. You can create empires. If you were to channel your dan tien's energy up to your solar plexus chakra, you would be able to manifest reality better. In your heart chakra, you would feel more love, etc. etc. etc.

Learn to direct this energy upwards into other chakras. You want to be more healthy, so, in this case, allow the energy to go into your heart and let it heal you. The affects of performing a dan tien meditation are enormous. You will feel more alive than you have ever felt. If you do the meditation long enough, the signs will begin to be experienced in the palms.

Your palms will heat up. At first, they will be warm, but they can progressively get so hot that they burn. They can even turn red. Strangely enough, the burning isn't painful, but, rather, it is exhilarating. You feel as though your palms are on fire, but the feeling is so amazing that you just want them to burn even more.

This was all of the sexual energy in your dan tien. You can use this energy in combat as well, but you need to become more adept with it. You need to learn how to truly harness this power. The dan tien is a pale orange chakra, and it is located three inches behind your abdomen, as stated before.

The Dan Tien Chakra Meditation

The dan tien is a pale orange chakra; therefore, when you are meditating, visualize all the important components to be pale orange.

1. Close your eyes, and take in a deep breath while slowly counting to four.

2. Exhale for a count of four, rest your arms on your lap, cross your legs, and hold your hands in such a way that your right fingers rest on your left fingers, and your thumbs rest on top of each other, creating a big circle. Let this rest in front of your abdomen.

3. Place the tip of your tongue to the roof of your mouth, and keep it as such for the duration of the exercise. Keep your mouth closed, and only breathe through your nose.

4. Repeat this breath cycle as such for 30 cycles. What this will do is get your mind and body into synchronization. This is absolutely important, because this is one of the beginning stages of feeling the oneness of the universe.

5. Breathe in, and visualize a flat, pale orange, disc right below your sternum, behind your solar plexus. The flat side of this disc is facing forward instead of facing the ceiling. Visualize, and feel, pale orange orbs of energy going through your nostrils and flowing straight into your dan tien chakra. As you are inhaling, also allow pale orange energy from the universe to vortex into the dan tien chakra directly through your abdomen.

6. Let the energy gather there. When you exhale, visualize, and FEEL, that the dan tien chakra is spinning clockwise. It is spinning slowly.

7. Repeat steps five and six for the next 20 minutes, but let the chakra spin faster upon every exhale. Make sure the inhales and exhales are both the same duration and length as they were at the beginning of the exercise.

Chapter 19

The Root

This is the final chakra we are going to discuss. The root chakra is also a very important chakra- all seven are, because if one of them goes out of alignment, it really affects your whole life. This chakra allows you to feel a deep connection to the Earth. It allows you to stay grounded. It deals with security of nature.

This allows you to survive, and it causes you to be more animalistic. When your root chakra is awake, you begin to move without thought. You just *do* things. When you do these things, you are in alignment with the universe. You feel the flow of the universe exist within your body, and you feel as though you can fight with its power.

The root chakra allows you to feel secure, and it really makes you serene and calm. You truly feel as though you are a part of this universe, and that the great mother is always here to nurture you and protect you. It may seem as though this is one of the weaker chakras, but you are mistaken.

When someone's root chakra is strong, not even lightning can uproot that person. Nobody can push him or her down. There are martial artists who have evolved this chakra so much that seven people can push on them, and they will not budge. When you are rooted, you are more easily able to take attacks (both physical and psychological) and redirect their energy into the Earth itself so you are not harmed.

Disease, like I said earlier, is triggered, if not totally caused by, stress. When your root chakra is strong, you can simply redirect anything that would irritate you. You just channel it back into the Earth. Furthermore, you really feel so secure that nobody will want to harm you. Your victim mentality is gone. Where the solar plexus teaches you how to manifest, the root chakra teaches you how to be steadfast. It teaches you stability. It teaches you certainty.

Lastly, a strong root chakra can even show you your life's mission here on Earth. This chakra is located near the anus, and its color is pale red.

The Root Chakra Meditation

The Solar Plexus is a pale yellow chakra; therefore, when you are meditating, visualize all the important components to be pale yellow.

1.   Close your eyes, and take in a deep breath while slowly counting to four.

2.   Exhale for a count of four, rest your arms on your lap, cross your legs, and hold your hands in such a way that your right fingers rest on your left fingers, and your thumbs rest on top of each other, creating a big circle. Let this rest in front of your abdomen.

3.   Place the tip of your tongue to the roof of your mouth, and keep it as such for the duration of the exercise. Keep your mouth closed, and only breathe through your nose.

4.   Repeat this breath cycle as such for 30 cycles. What this will do is get your mind and body into synchronization. This is absolutely important, because this is one of the beginning stages of feeling the oneness of the universe.

5.   Breathe in, and visualize a flat, pale red, disc right below your sternum, behind your solar plexus. The flat side of this disc is facing forward instead of facing the ceiling. Visualize, and feel, pale red orbs of energy going through your nostrils and flowing straight into your root chakra. As you are inhaling, also allow pale red energy from the universe to vortex into the root chakra directly.

6.   Let the energy gather there. When you exhale, visualize, and FEEL, that the root chakra is spinning clockwise. It is spinning slowly.

7.   Repeat steps five and six for the next 20 minutes, but let the chakra spin faster upon every exhale. Make sure the inhales and exhales are both the same duration and length as they were at the beginning of the exercise.

Chapter 20

Resonance

Now that the chakras have been talked about, it is important that you learn about their impact on the world as a whole. There is a concept known as resonance. As you know, this universe acts on vibration. Absolutely everything is energy. This passage serves to teach you how everything harmonizes.

When you have enough crickets in a field, they will first chirp off beat. Eventually, they will chirp in unison. When you are in an audience, all it takes is for one person to clap in order to the whole audience to start clapping.

If you want to turn a good man bad, all you have to do is place that man in a group of hoodlums for a period of 30 days. At the end of those 30 days, the man will be so changed that he will seem like a completely different person.

This is resonance. Basically, in a field of energy, like always attracts like. When there is a strong current, its power must be matched. If the power cannot be matched, the current will eventually dissipate.

All things live in such a balance. Now as far as chakras and resonance go, there is something known as the Maharishi Effect. This principle states that when a bunch of people with high vibrations who meditate come together to meditate in unison, it raises the consciousness of the world.

As a matter of fact, you yourself a raising the consciousness of this world simply because you are reading this book. Whenever you engage in any activity that strengthens your faith, your belief, your soul, your heart, and your energetic faculties, it raises the vibration of the world.

In Dr. David Hawkins' masterpiece *Power vs. Force*, he essentially teaches us that the world is composed of varying levels of consciousness. In his book, he teaches us that consciousness exists in levels of 1 to1000. In order for us to have life, we need to be operating at levels of 200 or more. Below 200, you experience disease.

Level 1000 is a VERY rare level of consciousness, and only a few people have ever achieved it. Jesus, Buddha, and Thoth were amongst the few. These there men were all capable of shifting reality in ways most people cannot fathom, not even myself. I am nowhere near the level of these three. My consciousness just hasn't risen to that degree.

Jesus was able to bring the dead back to life, he was able to walk on water, he was able to turn water into wine. Buddha was able to burn holes through walls with his eyes when he meditated. He was able to heal people with his energies as well. Thoth taught us writing. He was an immortal. He would meditate in the mantel of the Earth in what he called the Halls of Amenti for 50 year stretches in order to keep his youth. He is hailed on many Egyptian pyramids.

Interestingly enough, all three men have faced symbolic deaths. When Jesus "died", he was resurrected back on the third day. The Buddha was poisoned to death, but he also was spotted alive a few days after. As the story goes, a passerby noticed the Buddha walking with one sandal on his foot. The stranger knew the Buddha had recently died, so he could not believe what he was seeing. Later on, he went to exhume the Buddha's body, and when he saw what was in the grave, it confirmed his insanity: there was nothing but one sandal.

Thoth apparently just voluntarily left the world. He ascended to a higher realm, and he said that he would come back when he desires to, as Drunvalo Melchizedek states in his book *The Flower of Life: Part 1*.

The Buddha, Jesus, and Thoth taught many similar teachings, and they all expressed love. All this rivalry and hate needs to end. Let's take for instance something taken directly from The Emerald Tablets of Thoth.

> "As above, so below. As within, so without." Thoth is teaching us that the world is just a reflection of your thoughts, and that there is no external world independent of the world within us.

> Buddha talked about nirvana, and he said, "Every human is the author of his own health or disease."

> In John 10:22-39, Jesus says *"Is it not written in your Law, `I have said you are gods'?"*

> In Luke 17:20-21, it is said that *"The kingdom of God cometh not with observation; neither shall they say, Lo*

here! or, Lo there! For behold, the kingdom of God is within you. (Luke 17:20-21)

In the Jewish tradition of the Talmud, it states *"We do not see things as they are. We see things as we are."*

The wars of the world, the hatred, and the malice all have to end. We are all fighting for the same message. How we express that message may vary according to religion and belief, but the message is still the same. We are all love, and we all came from love.

Science and spirituality are coming together at alarming rates. With advances in scientific knowledge, we are now realizing that the universe exists on batches of energy, and that everything is a movement of consciousness.

You must begin to now see that we are not separate beings, but rather, we are powerful components of a huge ocean. The universe is just one great ocean. Your actions and thoughts are felt absolutely everywhere. Be careful of your dreams and intentions, because they will be felt across the universe. You are a beacon of power.

Your whole life, you have been focusing on the wrong things. People who are unhealthy focus on disharmonic health. FOCUS your attention on what you WANT. You might think that focusing on what you want is selfish and that others might get hurt along the way. You might be thinking that people need to be *realistic*. Well, let me ask you something: HOW realistic are YOU being by constantly stating that absolutely everything in your life is horrible? You can read this book, and not many people in most countries can even afford such a luxury. You live in the most powerful time in human history, and you still decide to be a pessimist? How realistic are *you*? Get over it. Life is beautiful, and you have to start seeing that. You need to shift your perception and think in terms of what you desire.

With resonance, realize that absolutely everything is a harmony. Every time you meditate, the world meditates with you. Every time you cry, the world cries with you. Every time you smile, the world smiles back. Every thought you have becomes manifest at the quantum level, at a level below the quark, possibly. The thing is, it lasts for JUST a fraction of a second. Your thoughts need momentum, so the thoughts you think about MOST give the universe fuel for you to create more of what you are focusing on.

Jesus told the world that we could do all that he could, and more. Moses split the red sea. These seem like miracles in modern science, but they are actual events absolutely anyone can influence if they believe.

At the level of 1000, whatever you think about instantly manifests. You are truly awake, and you live between both realms of physical and ethereal reality. Before I talk about the realms, I must address more of this consciousness phenomenon.

Level 600 is where you should aim to reach in this life time. This is the level of pure love. Mother Theresa was at 600. Those who reach such a level truly awaken the world. According to Dr. Hawkins' research, most peoples' consciousness raises by only five points in their lifetimes; therefore, most healthy people operate at a level of roughly 205 or so. People dislike change.

If you hang around the wrong people, it will certainly have a bad affect on your being. If you flood your senses with visuals of slaughter and rape, your level of consciousness will plummet. Disease LOVES people with consciousness levels below 200, because disease cannot live in people, because they are easiest to infect. People at the level of 600 or more cannot be inflicted by disease.

Through meditation, you can raise you consciousness. Through reading the right books, you can raise your consciousness. You can pray, if you believe in God. If you do not believe in God, you can still spread love in whichever way you know how. The beauty a bout love is that you do not need to have faith in something outside of yourself in order to feel it.

Chapter 21

Hands-on Healing

It is very important that you practice the meditations prescribed earlier, specifically the dan tien meditation. As you can tell, this book is getting more and more mystical as we continue. Thank you for sticking around! Hopefully, you have been practicing everything as we're moving along. It is very important to adopt the strategies lain within this book to achieve the fullest effect of health.

What we are going to speak about next is a very practical approach towards healing. This is a very special chapter, because it involves others as well. You will be able to heal yourself and others within tangible distance. You will also be able to heal others who are not close to you.

You are probably wondering how this is at all possible, but you shouldn't be too confused or surprised at this point, because we have been talking about quantum mechanics and energies throughout the entire scope of this book thus far.

Remember that energy always flows where attention goes. There is a very, very, large system of healing, and it is considered an art form. Reiki is a Japanese art that focuses on using the palms, instead of medicine, to heal a patient. Dr. Richard Gordon's book Quantum Touch focuses entirely on this art.

The subject, alone, can reach excesses of thousands of pages. There is the practice of acupuncture which focuses on placing needles on various meridians of the body. There is the practice of acupressure which focuses on healing a body through massage. The Chinese have special herbal remedies, many of which are illegal in most parts of the world due to their effectiveness, called Dit Da Jow.

This passage focuses on the basics of healing, but, do not take these basics lightly. What you have to do is first realize that the universe completely acts on vibration. Realize that everything is harmonic. When you raise your vibration, as Dr. Gordon teaches, other vibrations around you must also match. Really high vibrations are contagious, and they lift lower vibrations immediately. In other words, you could think of how contagious enthusiasm is. Love really puts a smile on peoples' faces.

What you must do now is learn to circulate your chi, your energy, through your body. I suggest that you spend a few minutes doing the breathing cycles for the dan tien. Let yourself really feel the chi heat up your palms.

Now, let's change things up. Before, when you were exhaling, you were just causing the dan tien to spin faster. Now, upon every exhale, allow the chi to escape the dan tien and travel upwards to your shoulders, down your arms, and into your palms. When you inhale, gather more chi into your abdomen. When you exhale, exhale the chi back into your palms. This practice teaches you how to channel your energy through your body.

Practice, Practice, Practice! Energy circulation is very, very easy. You can experience results within seconds. Keep your attention on your palms the entire time. Allow yourself to feel the amazing presence of the moment.

Understand that energy can absolutely be channeled. Matter of fact, according to Newtonian physics, that is exactly how things work. Energy is always transferred from one object to another when they make contact. Anytime you hit somebody, that person receives your energy.

What you are doing now is consciously sending another person, or yourself, energy. It is very invigorating to practice on another person. Find somebody who is hurting, and touch an area of that person's body. You see, if there is anybody in pain, it is because that person is out of harmony. When you raise your frequency and vibration, you make it so that the person you are healing must also raise his or her frequency or vibration. As long as you focus on your vibration, the healing must occur.

Touch that person's area of pain, and focus on the healing. Send love. If you can, meditate while touching that person. Breathe in the energy through your dan tien, send it up to your shoulders, down your palms, and straight into the person. The person will start to feel better if you keep it up. Now, this pain relief could possibly be just temporary, because, as I stated earlier, all pain comes from the mind. You might be giving this person temporary relief, because the true root of this pain is in something else entirely. A week down the road, the person you healed may have the same problem all over again. In any case, all sorts of healing are harmonious. You can use this application to heal broken bones, skin disorders, rashes, heart problems, and much, much, more.

When your skill advances, you will be able to see results instantaneously. It's quite an interesting phenomenon that you are going to have to test out and see for yourself in order to fully grasp the concept.

In order to be in the absolute best position to be able to heal at any given moment in time, I suggest that you practice for at least a half hour every single day in order to get yourself into prime shape. If you do this, there is no telling what you will be able to do. You will be able to command energy directly. You will feel unstoppable, and you will be able to heal.

At more advanced stages, you will be able to heal with all of your chakras. I would suggest that you heal with your heart chakra and dan tien together to get an even greater effect. Practice makes perfect. Focus on one chakra for now. As your skill increases, you will be able to add more to your repertoire.

Distance healing requires more concentration, because you are not healing yourself or someone in your tangible proximity. This requires a lot of focus and concentration. You really have to feel the connection between you and the person you are healing.

What you do is close your eyes and see that person in front of you as if he or she were actually there. You heal that residual image of the person. As you do this, the person will begin to feel the healing take place in reality. Group healing sessions work extremely well for this. If you were to get about ten people into a room with the expectation to heal someone far away, results would be miraculously quick.

The reason for this is that you are building a mastermind , and when you build a mastermind, consciousnesses merge. When you have multiple consciousnesses focused on one goal, a brain network is made. With this brain network, you can accelerate the healing process like nothing else. Raise consciousness! Spread love!

Chapter 22

The Aura

We are now beginning to enter into higher faculties of existence. We spoke about quantum mechanics, chakras, healing, the mind, the patterns of belief, and we gave specific exercises for various uses. If you have been doing everything in this book as it has been prescribed so far, you should be slowly turning into a maverick of the healing arts. As we move on, things are going to get even wilder.

You see, your aura and chakras are heavily related. There is a reason for the colors given to the chakras mentioned earlier, because these are also the major colors of your aura. Your aura is a field of energy that surrounds your body. It is, in many respects, a shield. It keeps anything that is not relevant to you away from you. At the very basic stages of aura reading, you will not see an aura at all.

What we want to do is first strengthen the third eye. Make sure you strengthen this chakra. This will help you clearly see auras. The reason why aura reading is important is that a person gives off many vibes. When you can read a person's aura, you are able to understand what kind of troubles he or she is facing. You see, disease is caused by imbalance. I have said this many, many times. If you can see the emotional or chakra imbalance a person is experiencing, you can more readily assess the situation.

When you are training to see auras, it can be a very difficult process at first. Just hang in there, and you will get the hang of it. It takes practice. What you want to do is first stare around your fingertips while taking your eyes slightly off center. You will eventually see a transparent wave of energy around the fingers. This wave emanates out of every single person's body.

As you train to see with your third eye, you will begin noticing colors. As you notice these colors, you will be more readily able to heal that person. The different colors you see pertain to the different chakras. Therefore, if you see a strong red wave, it means that the person feels connected and secure. If you see a rising of orange, it means sexual thoughts. If you see green, it means pure love, and etc.

Your aura is affected by every single thought that occurs in your mind. When you think of a negative thought, your aura weakens. Conversely, when your thoughts are positive, your aura strengthens. When you are feeling very positive feelings, your emanates those feelings into the universe. Remember when we talked about the akka strings earlier? These akka strings are connected to your aura.

Interestingly enough, people who have diseases or are very susceptible to diseases have very weak auras. Their defenses are down, and they are constantly in the wrong vibration. It's absolutely wonderful to be able to see auras, because you get to really know what states of emotion a person is in. It's like staring into a person's soul and being able to figure out what makes that soul up.

It is very difficult to see auras at first. You should practice by viewing people against white backgrounds. You could start with your fingers. You could also do this at a bookstore, or just about anywhere. Don't look directly at the person. Just look a bit off focus, and you will see the transparent waves. As you train your third eye to awaken more and more, you will begin seeing the colors you need to see.

Practice hard, and you will absolutely see results. What's fascinating about being able to read auras is that you are also able to read energy signatures. Aura reading is the first step towards being able to correctly predict events. You see, we must not speak of the world in terms of future or past, because there is no such thing. All that exists is energy. If you can read energy, you can tell in which direction it is going. ALL events have energy trails leading up to them.

You can use this knowledge to know whether someone in *your* house is suicidal. You can see someone's aura and know whether the heart is on the verge of decaying, or whether there is something wrong with the prostate, or the throat, etc. etc. Being able to read auras gives you the power of foresight so that you can prevent something dangerous from occurring. It's a very valuable tool.

Chapter 23

The Higher Realms

The universe exists on vibration, as you already know. There are many cosmic forces at play that cannot detect because we are not in their vibration. Dog whistles, for instance, are at such high pitches that our ears cannot detect them. Ultraviolet rays are also invisible to the human eye. In such a manner, there is far more to the universe that we have either yet to observe or are unable to. I forget where I learned this, but apparently all of that we can see, hear, smell, taste, touch, and experience only accounts for 4% o the universe. There is a whopping 96% that remains "missing"!

You see, when you are at a certain vibration, you can only see things that are in your vibration. You can only see things that are in your alignment. Everything else is gone. When you are depressed, all you see is sadness. Even if happiness were to walk up to you and say hello, you would not see it because you are lost in the depths of your despair.

As such, there are higher realms that exist. The physical realm is the realm we are most inclined to seeing; however, higher than flesh and bone are realms of existence that are constantly "watching us" while they stay invisible to us. The biggest realm that surrounds us is the ethereal realm, and it dominates our physical realm.

In the realms around us, there is conscious network of energies and vibrations that are so high that our physical senses cannot detect them. We have to allude to a sixth sense in order to understand such phenomena. This is why you were taught the chakra exercises earlier.

According to Robert Bruce's *Astral Dynamics*, peoples' souls are connected to their bodies by something called the silver cord. When we go to sleep, our souls- or, you may say "consciousnesses"- step outside of our bodies. We are able to access our physical bodies upon waking because we are still connected via the silver cord. When we die, this silver cord is severed.

One of your greatest fears is probably death. Your worries of death have probably taken the best of you, and you might be, as a result, worrying yourself to death. You probably fear that there may be no afterlife after your stay on Earth. If you do believe in an afterlife, you probably are afraid that it will be a place of confusion and chaos.

Scientific studies have been conducted to show otherwise. Studies are now being done that are beginning to prove that (1), an afterlife does exist, and (2), it is quite blissful to die. Dr. Sam Parnia, according to Time Magazine, "is one of the world's leading experts on the scientific study of death." Parnia has been studying what happens to us when we die. What doctors who study death are really studying are near death experiences.

An NDE occurs when a patiently is clinically proven dead and then is resuscitated back to life. According to Dr. Jeffrey Long's book *Evidence of the Afterlife*, patients who experience an NDE have a life altering event. In many cases, they are fully conscious of what is going on in the hospital room as the doctors try to bring them back to life. When a person is clinically proven dead, his or her consciousness is gone; therefore, it should be impossible for any details to be perceived by the deceased. When the deceased is resuscitated back to life, he or she can tell everything that happened during the procedure. Many times, those who have NDE's can even see what is going on beyond the room.

A great pattern many NDE's convey is that when the person dies for that short period of time, there is usually bright light. Upon death, there is a heavenly love that shines down, and everything is beautiful. The experience is so addicting, so amazing, that many wish that they never came back to their Earth bodies after returning back to life. Upon death, they are met with deceased relatives. The relatives are never old. Those who experience NDE's are usually given a decision as to whether or not they want to go back to Earth. There is no bias in the decision, and no emotion. The soul can choose to stay or to go back. The second a decision is made, the decision is final. Those who come back have a reawakening. They never fear death any longer, and their lives are completely revitalized.

According to the book, near death experiences teach us that there really is a life after this life. The life is far more beautiful, and this life dulls in comparison. It's amazing what science can do these days.

Chapter 24

The Man Who Laughed Himself out of Cancer

This book is about the cures of diseases, and now it is very important that we focus on actual things you can do to make yourself feel better and get rid of sickness. Many say that "laughter is the best medicine". So much focus is placed on negativity and stress that nobody talks about positive emotions. Studies have shown that disease can be triggered by stress. Newer studies show that positive energy can cause the body to actually heal. Laughter is one of the most positive emotions we can emit. When we are laughing, we are feeling joyful. Our bodies are bursting with energy when we laugh, and everything feels wonderful.

But, how can laughter cure us? What effect can laughter have on the body whatsoever? These are all questions that we are going to take into consideration now. A positive emotion, according to Dr. David Hawkins in his book *Power vs. Force*, is exponentially stronger than a negative emotion. Matter of fact, it seems as though the universe itself is based on positive energy. According to Stephen Hawking,

> There are something like ten million million million million million million million million million million million million million million (1 with eighty zeroes after it) particles in the region of the universe that we can observe. Where did they all come from? The answer is that, in quantum theory, particles can be created out of energy in the form of particle/antiparticle parts. But that just raises the question of where the energy came from. The answer is that the total energy of the universe is exactly zero. The matter in the universe is made out of positive energy. (generationterrorists)

The universe was founded on positive energy. Why must we be different? I am reminded of an amazing story of a man who literally laughed himself out of sickness. Briefly put, Norman Cousins was a man who, in 1964, was diagnosed with a spinal tissue degenerative disease. Doctors said he wouldn't make it. Cousins was determined to get healthy at any cost. He felt that the atmosphere of a hospital was too gloomy and depressing, so he decided to take things into his own hands. He began thinking that stress and negative emotions can cause disease, and if this is the case, then perhaps positive emotions could do the exact opposite. He thought that there could be a possibility that positive emotions could heal disease (TheHealingPowerofLaughter.Blogspot.com). Instead of moping around, he decided to just watch some funny movies. He grabbed a bunch of hysterical movies, and he burst out laughing for long stretches of time. Amazingly, his pain would go away, and he would fall asleep like a baby. The next day, he would repeat the procedure. In this way, his body began to naturally heal itself. Eventually, he was admitted back into work, and the rest is history.

Laughter truly is very powerful medicine. You can use it to heal wounds simply because of your intense focus on the positive energy you are emitting. Remember how we talked about positive energies earlier? When your focus is on positive feelings, you emanate positive feelings into the universe.

Today, go out and watch some funny movies. Go see a standup show. Do something that makes you laugh. Really get into the habit of laughing. People don't laugh enough. Laughter is contagious, and it is incredibly healthy for the immune system and the body.

Be careful not to laugh at someone else's expense or misfortune. This is very cruel, and it will not lift your spirit like healthy laughter would. Make it a point to laugh every single day in order to get the maximum impact. Go out and laugh!

Chapter 25

Alkalinity and pH

This is something you pretty much already know to be true. I will provide some scientific background to it, and then I will teach you how to live according to this lifestyle. Alkalinity and acidity are a part of the pH scale. This scale ranges from 0 to 14. Numbers closer to 0 are more acidic, and numbers closer to 14 are more basic (the substance acts as a base). The more basic a substance is, the more alkalinity that substance has.

The universe loves balance, so it's not surprising that neutrality exists at a pH of 7, and water is at 7. You want to always be in harmony with your forces; therefore, realize that if your body is either too acidic or too basic, you are destined for doom.

When your body is too close to 1 or 14, you are in a very dangerous zone, and you could even die if you stay in this region long enough. Optimally, and you should always strive for optimal health, you want to be around 6.5 and 7.5

You can test your body's pH in three main ways: you can do a blood test, a urine test, and a saliva test. The list goes in order of effectiveness; therefore, the blood test is the most accurate, but it is also the most difficult to assess, the urine is very easy and much more accurate than saliva, and the saliva test is what you should use as a last resort because its numbers are nowhere near as accurate at the first two tests.

You can buy pH test strips and apply your urine to them to get a nice indicator as to what your body's pH is. Now, the ideal area you want to be, of course, is at a 7. Most people live very acidic lifestyles. They eat things that deteriorate their bodies, so if they were to amp up by eating a load of basic materials, they would not be putting their bodies into danger at all.

People are just too acidic! Most likely, if your test fails, your test will indicate a number less than 6.5 If this is the case, it means your body is too acidic, and you need to make some changes. Now, there have been volumes of literature written on this subject. Feel free to read all you need to read about this subject; however, realize that you do not need to become too attached to the subject matter. There is no need to make a mountain out of a mole hill.

The things your grandmother taught you when you were young still apply today. Eat lots of fresh vegetables, drink lots of water, and eat lots of fruit. You should also cut down on your meat intake, because meat is very acidic. If you like meat, always make sure you balance it out by eating a lot more greens. The rule of thumb is that only 1/4th of your plate should consist of meat, whereas the other 3/4th consists of healthy greens.

- Examples of Alkaline Foods:
    - Pumpkin, green beans, flowers, apples, grapes, oranges, peaches, bananas, whey protein powder (awesome for body builders!), walnuts, chestnuts, onions, nightshade, lettuce, berries, watermelons, raw almonds.
- Examples of Acidic Foods:
    - All kinds of meat, all rice, oats, oatmeal, spaghetti, black beans, kidney beans, butter, ice cream, milk, blueberries, corn, cranberries, beer, soda, peanut butter.

Now, we are not talking about cutting out acidic foods completely. In order for your body to be healthy, you need acids; however, most diets these days are so acidic that bodies are being torn apart. If you are going to have acidic food, make sure you neutralize all of the acidity with foods that are more alkaline. This balance is a harmony between positrons and electrons. Positrons are acidic, and electrons are negative. It's like yin and yang all over again! Once the energies balance out, you have harmony.

Your actionable for today is to go out and buy some pH test strips from your local pharmacy. Test out your acid-alkaline levels, and then adjust your diet as seen fit. Add more greens to your diet. Just by doing this, alone, you will see a drastic drop in your weight because your body will stop clinging onto your fat.

Chapter 26

Magnetic Therapy

As you are **well** aware now, the universe is energy. Electrons are drawn to magnetism. Without getting too scientific here, let's talk about what magnetic therapy is.

Your body consists of many metals, and your blood is abundant with iron. Iron is easily drawn to magnets. Your blood also has heavy stores of chi in it, and when your blood goes to a wounded area, that area begins to get healed. The reason for this is that your blood carries many nutrients within it, and these nutrients must be exported to every single area of your body in order for you to live.

When a magnet is applied to certain parts of your body, it helps direct more blood flow to those regions, thus causing quicker rates of healing. You need a very strong magnetic to feel the effects; therefore, it is best for you to use a neodymium rare earth magnet. These can be bought quite cheaply, and they do absolute wonders.

They are extremely powerful, and they should be kept away from electronics. Dropping just one of these small magnets (they can be half the size of a quarter, and just as thin) on a hard drive can fully erase everything and kill the machine upon impact.

Earth itself has magnetic energy, and according go Gregg Braden in his book *Fractal Time: The Secret of 2012 and a New World Age*, this magnetic energy is Earth's heart beat. The magnetic pull, at one point, had a rating of 4.0, and life flourished in such a state of magnetic energy. Over the last 100 years, due to soil erosion and poisons being emptied into our foods, the ratio has drastically dropped to a .4. When soil is magnetic crops grow quicker and more safely.

Therefore, there is a substantially positive effect on magnets when it comes to growth and healing. You should make it a point to sleep on magnetic mattresses, wear magnetic bracelets when you sleep, and do your best to have magnets directing your blood flow absolutely whenever you possible.

Now, because magnetic living can become a bit expensive, you do not necessarily have to go out and buy something today. This book was written in a way as to give you the most affordable lifestyle change you can make. If you have the money, I urge you to buy the magnetic healing equipment. You spend $1/3^{rd}$ of your life in bed. Why not get something that will possibly even increase your life by another third?

Today's actionable is your calling: choose to buy something that can prolong your life, or you can hold out. If you do absolutely everything else stated in this book and totally disregard this, your life will still face a massive transformation. It really is your call, though.

Chapter 27

Your Diet

The way you eat influences everything. First things first, you must look at your metabolism. A healthy body always has a nice rate of metabolism. Your body must be able to burn food into energy quickly, and it must get rid of any excesses it does not need. In order to best aide the body in the process of metabolism, we must learn to eat intelligently.

Instead of having three large meals, you need to have six smaller meals. Filling your body up in large doses does nothing but slow you down. Instead, take smaller sizes of your meals and eat only until you are satisfied. There is no need in filling your stomach. There is no need to get bloated.

Make sure you ALWAYS have breakfast. You were sleeping the entire night, and your body had no food. Breakfast is the way getting your body into action. Do not skip it. Your diet should be balanced, and it should consist of healthy grains, proteins, vegetables, fruits, fats, oils, and water.

Avoid junk food as much as you can, because it has no nutritional value for you. If you are trying to overcome a sickness, this **especially** applies to you. Why make matters worse by giving your body garbage to run on?

- Essential Oils
  - Flax Seed Oil.
  - Olive Oil
  - Primrose Oil
  - Omega 3 Fish Oil
  - Krill Oil

- Nuts:
  - Walnuts
  - Cashews
  - Legumes
  - Peanuts
  - Pecans
- Meats
  - Fish
  - Chicken
  - Turkey
  - Eggs
  - Duck

You should have a variety of foods from this list. Try to avoid pork and red meat, because they are detrimental to your health. Flax seed oil is an absolute must if you want to be at optimum levels of health. Don't fry your oils, because that can make your oil toxic. Add lots of fruits and vegetables to your diet as well.

Make sure you get your daily intake of vitamins too. It would be a great idea to get whole food vitamins, because they are much healthier than normal vitamins, but they are also more expensive. If you can't afford whole food vitamins, then take normal vitamins.

Multivitamins are the best way to go if you want to get your whole dosage in one shot. The absolute best thing you can do is completely avoid supplements altogether and get your nutrients from food; however, this can be very expensive. If you can afford it, I would tell you to just go for it 100% and get all of your nutrients from food.

When speaking in terms of efficiency, however, it is still awesome to take your vitamins in the form of tablets. You should be taking in as many fruits and vegetables as you possibly can. Now, there are also capsulated greens which you can take to help aide yourself into recovery, but actual food is always best!

Make sure you are constantly feeding yourself throughout the day. You should have six small meals, and you should sneak on fruits, nuts, veggies, and other healthy food between meals throughout the day. The rule of thumb is that you should be eating something every 2-3 hours.

Try to avoid enriched carbs at all cost. White breads and processed grains have almost no nutritional value. When you eat these substances, you are, for lack of a better word, loading yourself up with cardboard. Whole wheat is a much better alternative.

All in all, you need to watch your diet. There is nothing "new" in this section that you don't already know. You need to make changes in your life, and diet is a huge factor in your health. If you are destroying your body by eating all of the wrong foods, how can you expect yourself to become fully healthy? I did talk about belief systems earlier, but I also believe that God helps those who make an effort to help themselves. You have to take action.

Go out and buy yourself some multivitamins and some essential oils for now. Don't worry about the fruits, vegetables, and meat until you read the rest of this book. If you are motivated to buy some healthy alternatives, then go for it! Don't go too crazy on your spending, but go out and buy something to spice up your kitchen. If you can't afford to buy anything right now, at least get rid of the junk food that's rotting away in your kitchen. The next time you decide to buy a bag of chips, buy some bananas instead.

Watch what you eat.

Chapter 28

Exercise

Exercise is absolutely important for your health. If you are not getting at least 30 minutes of exercise a day, you are looking forward to a life of ills and aches. Now, before you partake in any rigorous exercise, it is best that you consult your doctor. If you are able to exercise, then start now. You should be moving every single day. You may ride bikes, swim, hike, fish, run, or anything else that gets you moving. Just move! One great example is running.

Running pumps your blood quickly through your body, it makes your lungs strong, it makes your heart strong, and it does many other things that are so beneficial to your health that entire books have been written on the subject. If you dislike running, start by walking. Walk for 30 minutes and keep your heart pumping. If weight loss is your goal, you need to have a constant heart beat of a little over 130 beats per second for at least 30 minutes. If you run too quickly, your body won't burn any fat. If you walk, you won't really be making a dent in your physique. Jogging is the way to go for weight loss.

You also need to be lifting weights periodically throughout the week. You should aim for a minimum of 3 times per week in order to keep your muscles from atrophying. Remember, if you don't use it, you lose it! Combine diet with exercise in order to get the full effect.

The truth is, many diseases can spring just by you living a sedentary lifestyle. When you don't exercise, toxins build up in your body. If you are sick, it makes recovery even worse. Now, there are different levels of sickness. If you are terribly sick, exercise can possibly worsen the issue. This is why it is best to consult a doctor beforehand; however, if all you have is a cold, there is no reason to avoid working out.

If you combine exercise with everything else in this book, it will absolutely speed up your recovery like nothing else. Bodies in motion stay in motion.

Chapter 29

Your Social Circle

Pay CLOSE attention, because this is potentially the most important chapter you will read. The only reason I did not place it earlier in the book is that I wanted you to first become totally self empowered before you decided to expand your social circle. When you start with the self, the right people start to align up. I truly believe that. When you have a desire, and you hold fast to a belief, when you send out a vibration, you are matched to the right situations and events.

Your social circle is absolutely important. There is a rule in psychology called the law of five. Basically, if I want to know how much money you make, all I have to do is ask your five best friends what their salaries are. If I average their salaries together, I can know exactly how much you make. You are the average of the five people you spend most time with.

This is why it is absolutely essential that you constructively choose your relationships. Only spend time with people who serve your purpose. If you hang around those who give you negative vibes, people who make you disbelieve, people who take you off track, you will be thrown off track yourself.

You have to live your life by design. Realize that there are OTHERS out there who have overcome hurdles. There are others out there who practice the law of attraction daily. There are others out there who are living a lifestyle consisting of healthy foods. If you want to become rich, hang out with wealthy people. If you want to become healthy, hang out with healthy people.

Your actionable is to find a place where people are focused on health and positivity. Check online for groups of people that are near your house. Join a gym. Join a success club. If you can't afford memberships, you have NO excuses to make. You can still go to your library and simply read books on success. You can go to websites filled with healthy people. You can join chat rooms and blogs. When your mind is constantly surrounded by health and success, THAT is exactly what you will get. Don't just stop at this book. You must make health a part of your life. Do it!

Chapter 30

The Fung Shui of your Environment

The Chinese really have hit a home run when it comes to energy. Not only have they mastered ways of healing the body, using energy for combat (this will not be discussed in this book), and healing people with touch, but they have also taught us how to organize our environments for optimum energy flow.

Feng shui (fung-shway) is the Chinese art of environmental energy flow. Basically, you could call it interior/exterior decorating with a splash of harmony. Your environment is a reflection of who you are, so are the people you hang out with (read the previous chapter AGAIN), and so are the object you place around yourself.

Now, I am not a feng shui artist by any stretch of the imagination, so I really can't teach you a whole lot about it. Just like everyone else, I have my flaws. This is one area I don't want to discuss too heavily, because I have much to learn about the art myself. The point I am driving you towards is that you must be careful about what you surround yourself with.

If your house is filled with gloomy pictures, depressing colors, and it is dirty, you must do something about it! If you don't have the money to buy better furniture, you should at least clean up your house. Take down posters of violence and ill disease. Your house is your soul's living quarters. Treat your quarters like a temple. Where you live is sacred.

If you have the money, buy better furniture. Hang up beautiful paintings. If you are crafty enough, you don't even have to spend a fortune! There are many garage sales filled with art that you can buy for less than a dollar. The point isn't WHERE you got your stuff from, the point is that you have it. Make your house as beautiful as you can possibly make it.

Take the television out of your BEDROOM. TAKE IT OUT! The bedroom should only be used for sleeping and for bonding. If you watch television, you might turn on programs that will negatively influence your mind. For your sake and mine, don't turn on the news. The news has made billions of dollars by telling you about all of the negative sides of the world. You don't need this. You are better than this.

If you really have the money, hire an interior decorator to give parts of your house a major up lift. You can also just buy plants and put them in various locations. Plant life always brings good energy.

Have nice, vibrant, colors in your house. If there are dark, gloomy, spots, paint them. This is a really "hands-on" section, but it will give you massive rewards in the end.

If your environment is beautiful, you will feel beautiful for being a part of it. When you feel well, all is well. Your actionable now is to do whatever you can to spice up your house. If all you can afford to do is clean, then clean it! Make your living place beautiful. Take the television OUTSIDE OF YOUR BEDROOM.

Do whatever you can to make your house look extremely beautiful today. There is a guest that's going to be coming in: the NEW, HEALTHY, you! Invite that person in with full passion and excitement.

Chapter 31

The Power of Water

You NEED to drink water. It is vital to your existence. It is common knowledge that 75% of your body is made of water. 2/3rd's of the world is also made of water. Water is important, yet so many people neglect drinking it. We live in a time when water is so easy to come by that people should be jumping at it; however, most people take for granted the luxuries they are handed to on a silver platter.

You need to be drinking at least half your body weight in ounces every single day in order to achieve a proper state of health. For many of you, dehydration is the only reason you are sick. When you drink water, your blood flows more easily through your veins. Your cells grow and die more quickly. Waste is exported through your body with far greater ease.

You feel younger, and you also look younger when you drink a lot of water. Toxins are washed out of your body. Your joints are lubricated, and your body functions perfectly. You wouldn't put soda into your car, would you? DON'T flood your body with soft drinks. One can of soda is so acidic that it takes about 32 glasses of water to neutralize the acidity. If you drink 8 glasses, that means it will still take you 4 days to achieve harmony. But, who drinks that much?! Who drinks 8 glasses a day? Most of us drink, perhaps, three pure glasses of water. The rest of our water comes from coffee, booze, soda, and juices.

So, let me reiterate what I said earlier: you need to drink at LEAST half your body weight in ounces of PURE water daily.

Your actionable for this entire week is to drink at least six glasses of water throughout the day. You can do it. People can get hung over, but they can't drink healthy doses of water? There are NO excuses for not following this actionable. Water is virtually free, it is everywhere, and if you can afford this book, you can surely afford six glasses of *free* water. Do it.

Chapter 32

Acupuncture/Acupressure

Acupuncture is the Chinese art of needle therapy. Your body has far more chakras than the seven listed in this book. There are hundreds, if not thousands, of chakras all over your energy body. The seven main ones are the most important; however, there are many more which must be taken into consideration.

The Chinese believe that all disease occurs due to blockages of energies in various meridians of the body. As discussed earlier, a meridian is the "vein" in which your chi flows. When one of the seven chakras are blocked, there can be tremendous problems in the body. When one of the smaller meridian points is blocked, there can be discomfort.

It is important to unblock all of these points. Acupressure is similar to acupuncture, except that it does not use needles. An acupressure specialist massages your body and loosens up energy blockages. This process is similar to the emotional freedom techniques (EFT) being plastered all over the internet. Essentially, when there is a blockage of energy, your flow is cut off, and you feel sick in that part of the body. Imagine not being able to get blood to a certain part of the body. That body part will begin to decay instantly. Now, apply this concept to the energy body. Your energy body can never decay, so it sends out signals of pain to your physical body to allow you to know that something is not right.

If you are in a great deal of pain or sickness, it might be a good idea to go seek out a specialist in either one, or both, of these areas. When your body's energy gates are open, you can feel the bliss of the universe flow through you.

Chapter 33

Yoga

Yoga's benefits to the body and mind are monumental. You are taught to do breathing exercises that unite the mind and body. Do you remember when we spoke earlier about the environment? We talked about how it is a reflection of ourselves.

Well, your body is also a reflection of your inner states. Your body is a representation of who you are inwardly. If you change your inner focus, your body will also change. If your body is inflexible, it could mean that your energy body is also rigid.

Yoga teaches your body how to be flexible. It teaches you patience. It teaches you how to relax even in the face of opposition. It's a spiritual ballet, and you get to really harness full control over your body.

Take a few yoga lessons. Your whole body, mind, health, and soul will be revitalized. There is great power in your life force, and that force is conducted through your breath. It's not important about which style of yoga you should pursue. Just go out there today and sign up for an introductory class.

It will do you wonders. When you practice yoga, you learn to rclax cvcry single muscle in your body. You truly become aware of your environment, and you start living in the present moment.

Your mind is free, and you are able to think more clearly. When your mind is under you control, you get to more easily focus on the things you DO want, as opposed to the things you do not want.

To get the full benefits, it is best to see an instructor; however, if you do not have the money, there still is NO excuse for you not to do yoga. You can go to YouTube and search up thousands of videos. If you have a Nintendo Wii, you can go out and buy a Wii Fit. There are over 25 yoga exercises in the Wii Fit alone, and they will truly make you stretch. Your local video rental store may have a section dedicated entirely to this. No excuses. Add yoga to your repertoire. Today, you are going to do at least 20 minutes of Yoga.

Follow the videos on YouTube. If a helicopter fell on your internet line, then go out to your local book store and buy some books. If you are strapped for cash, go to the library. If you are locked in a room, and the only thing you have is this computer, this book, and no internet connection, then stretch for 20 minutes.

You really have no way out of this. Take ACTION! If you had been doing everything in this book that I stated earlier, your mind and health should be so extraordinary that you will easily find an opportunity to practice yoga. Go, go, go!

Chapter 34

Giving to Others

One of the laws that run this universe is the law of giving. You really have to be a giver in this life. I learned a long time ago that in order for us to be successful, we must help other people become successful. We must truly give of ourselves to others in order to receive.

If you are strapped for cash, you still have no excuse. You need to stop being an excuse maker. If your mind is so focused on a lack of money, you will never make much of it anyway. Focus on what you WANT!

Anyway, become a giver. The BEST way to become a giver is by giving people something valuable that you have a lot of. Create value for others, and give to them something you have in abundance.

If all you have is a beautiful smile, then brighten up somebody's day by smiling at him or her. If you are a millionaire, then donate your cash to charities. If you are amazing at basketball, teach somebody how to play basketball- for free.

Sometimes, giving can come in the form of something sentimental such as attention. For instance, you can just lend someone your ear and listen to his or her story. You can tell people you love them. You can give hugs.

There is so much you can give, and if you would look for the goodness within you, you would see a wealth of abundance. Share that abundance with the world. If you want to get healthy, help somebody else get healthy. Feed your pet healthy food. Give your kids loving affection. Raise your plants well. You could even direct someone to this book!

I have respect for you, and I know you have ever intention to follow everything in this book. Well, now is your shot. Go give. I don't care if you have arthritis, cancer, syphilis, lupus, and are ten months behind on rent. There is something you have that can brighten up somebody else's day.

Live your life from the standpoint of creating value for others, and you will ALWAYS get value back. And, it is okay to want things back. You should expect to receive happiness and rewards for all that you give.

The universe loves givers, and givers are rewarded justly. Before you read this book, you probably came from a great place of negativity and self doubt. You probably felt as though you needed some hope, as though you needed a sign. I can understand that there was a point where you felt that you had absolutely no worth, that you were a victim caught in a storm of raging seas.

But now, the time of moping is over. You are better than that. Didn't we make a promise earlier that we would FIGHT through this? Well, now you have to fight to realize how wonderful you are. You came here for the truth, so there you have it. You have to change your vision and focus on creating value for others.

When you give to others, you feel abundant. It does not matter **what** you give. All that matters is that you give with love. And when you give love, love comes rushing back to you.

Make a list of all the great qualities you have. You must come up with at least 50 things. DO IT. This will cause you to stretch your mind and truly see you for how wonderful you are. Next, brighten up one person's day. You cannot move forward from this lesson until you have brightened up somebody's day.

DO NOT MOVE ON UNTIL YOU HAVE DONE THIS.

Chapter 35

Physical Contact

People are so afraid of expressing themselves. Men think that they should show no emotion. Women distance themselves from other women due to jealousy. All of this has to stop. We really need to feel the love. In the previous chapter, I talked about giving love. One of the best ways to give love to others is by touch.

When was the last time you hugged your loved ones? I'm not talking about fake hugs. Everyone has a fake hug. A fake hug is the one where you basically embrace each other with a five feet gap between your chests. A true hug is chest to chest, and it is completely felt. You can know the meaning of a hug by the feeling you get from it.

Women are quite touchy. Men are really lacking in this area. If you are a guy, you might just need some masculine energy. You might need to hug your father. You might need to play some football with your friends. You might want to play fight. Playing involves touch.

It's a shame that there are many people who die simply due to isolation. When you touch somebody, you acknowledge his or her presence. This chapter is short, but it is very, very, important.

You have to go out and give somebody a sincere hug today. It does not matter who. Just, go out and hug somebody. Hug that person with all of your heart.

Chapter 36

Live Your Life By Design

Many people die with regrets, because they did not live their lives out fully. Do not let this be you. When you have no direction in life, it causes you to look at stupid things and make yourself a victim towards them.

You start watching endless amounts of television, you spend time with the wrong people, you work at a job you hate, and your spirit is robbed of you. On your deathbed, you will feel as though you really could have done so much more if you had only tried.

Do not let this be you. You must now take charge of your life. These past 30+ days have been extraordinary, and your life has already reached new heights. You have been taking massive action towards a better life, and you deserve all the health the universe has to offer.

Now, it is time to bring the game to entirely different level. Take out your journal, and open up to a new page. What journal? The journal you've been writing in all this time, silly! Did you forget? You are supposed to have a journal! Now, let's continue.

On this new sheet of paper, make a heading that reads, "100 Goals I have achieved." Then, write down 100 goals you would like to achieve in this lifetime. The reason I have worded the heading as such as is that you are supposed to believe that you have already achieved the very thing you desire.

Go crazy. Write down everything you want. Write in terms of SPECIFICITY. Instead of writing that you want to be rich, write that you are millionaire/bi llionaire, or whatever you feel is rich. STOP. DO NOT even finish this chapter. GO NOW. Finish your list.

Okay, are you done?!

Great!

Now, your job is to take one item on your list into consideration and start taking action towards that item TODAY. If you want to be rich, then take action TOWARDS THAT.

If you want to lose weight, something you should have been doing as a result of reading this book anyway, GO FOR IT.

Your dreams are yours to conquer. So, go conquer them. Your life is yours now. When your mind is focused on a dream, sickness cannot touch you. Dream, and focus in terms of what you desire.

You MUST focus on what you desire. Now, Go!

Chapter 37

Homeopathic Medicine

This is a touchy area for me. I am not a doctor, so I cannot give medical advice. I want to explain what homeopathic medication is. Prescription drugs are ruining our bodies. My grandmother's death occurred because she was sick of taking medications for so many various ailments.

Realize that the prescription drug industry is a multibillion dollar industry, and there really isn't money in curing people. Cured people do not generate large revenues for insurance companies and doctors.

With that in mind, I still want you to continue taking whatever medication you are on, because I cannot make these decisions for you. What I will talk to you about is homeopathic medicine. You decide what you want.

Homeopathic medicine deals with vibrations. It was invented by the German physician, Samuel Hahnemann. He believed that when we are curing disease, we must apply various levels of vibration in order to get rid of it. Earlier we spoke of hands-on healing. This is the same concept, only it is in medicinal form. Hahnemann believed that if we diluted a substance enough, we would be left with its vibrational imprint instead. He would then capsulate that imprint and use it to treat patients.

I can't tell you to take an action step here. It is your call. It may be a good idea to look into homeopathic medications while you are taking your regular medications. Homeopathic medications have no side effects, so there is absolutely no harm in taking them. Due to FDA regulations, I cannot say that anything can cure anything other than a drug; therefore, realizing that all of this information is intended for entertainment, it could be beneficial to your life to switch to homeopathic medications. As long as your diet, mind, exercise, affirmations, and everything else is in tact, you should be experiencing such levels of bliss that you probably do not even need medication anymore. This is just food for thought.

Chapter 38

Healing through Music

Once again, the issue of environment comes into effect. We have to treat ourselves like temples! The music we listen to has a PROFOUND effect on our very beings. If we listen to uplifting music, our souls will be uplifted. Conversely, negative music can really harm our bodies.

We must constantly surround ourselves with models of excellence. Earlier, I spoke to you about your social circle. You are also greatly affected by the music you listen to. The music you listen to on a constant basis really can change your energetic signature. When your signature goes out of harmony, you fall sick.

I did not say this program was going to be easy. You really have to take charge of your life. You have to DEMAND excellence out of yourself. Some people listen to Gospels, others listen to Mozart, others listen to the Beatles. It does not matter what music it is, just as long as the music and lyrics from the heart.

Songs about killing, violence, destruction, murder, and drugs will take our bodies out of alignment to true health. When you are constantly flooded with this kind of information, you simply cannot help but to think in negative terms.

Now, I can't control your tastes in music. Music is one medium people are very attached to, and I can tell why. Music is beautiful. All that I ask for you to do is just try listening to twenty minutes of harmonic music today.

You could listen to meditation songs from YouTube, you could listen to The Beatles, some Explosions in the Sky, some Pachelbel, the Lord's music, and absolutely anything else that raises your soul's vibration. Just don't listen to anything that is violent or has negative connotations behind it.

Dr. Coldwell in Germany uses music to treat cancer patients, so realize that there is a great impact of music on your health.

Chapter 39

Energy Protection

There is energy all around us. There are negative thoughts and feelings all around us. One of the most potent forms of energy is electromagnetic. Cell phones, microwaves, and televisions all emit electromagnetic chaos energy. This energy can really cause disease and chaos in our lives. Years ago, this was a non issue because technology simply did not exist in the way it does today. Today, you can't avoid it. The energy is everywhere. If you keep your focus on what you want, if you focus on health, then the energy cannot harm you. However, it is always to be best protected.

You can buy Electromagnetic Chaos Eliminators, instruments that can be easily found through a Google search. They can come in the form of stickers, necklaces, and other variations.

Crystals are also very effective in collecting negative energy. If you buy a 24 quartz crystal, it can absorb negative energies from the environment and trap the energies within itself. There is a whole practice known as crystal therapy that goes beyond the scope of this book. There are gem stones and crystals that can be used to charge your chakras up, open up meridians, and they can even realign energy. Many exotic massage parlors use heated stones as ways of treating customers. Stones and crystals are also heavily involved in feng shui. A great example you encounter is in Japanese zen gardens. They make their gardens out of stone and sand in ways that are most harmonic with vibes of the universe.

There is great power in stones and crystals. Your actionable today is to go out and buy an electromagnetic chaos eliminator. It will be well worth your investment. You do not need to buy anything expensive. It's just always good to have great protection wherever you go. Your house should be the very first place you have harmony. However, when you go outside, it may be more difficult to keep control over your thoughts and feelings due to all the activities and noise. Your electromagnetic chaos eliminator, most preferably a necklace, will keep you sound and relaxed as you live your days out in the busy, busy world.

Chapter 40

Go Organic

Finally, we have reached our last chapter. I have saved this for last, because this is actually the most expensive procedure you can undergo. If you have the money for it, definitely take up opportunity to live such a lifestyle. Organic foods are the best foods you can eat.

Normal fruits, vegetables, and crops are loaded with pesticides. Pesticides are used to kill insects, and they can kill us as well. They harm the energetic structure of our food. Even food has an aura. Kirlian photography actually takes images of the energetic patterns around substances. Foods that pesticides sprayed over them have horrible energy structures. You can call these structures auras, because that's what they are.

Even our meat has horrible auras. First of all, our crops are loaded with pesticides. Secondly, many animals eat crops. Most animals are fed corn, something they shouldn't be eating anyway. Cows, for instance, are fed heavy amounts of corn because it makes them fatter. The problem is that this corn is flooded with pesticides, the cow's energy structure also gets destroyed because it isn't eating grass, and then we eat the cow. Meat, by the way, raises our acidity levels, and corn boosts that acidity even more.

There is a huge cycle of chaos going on here. In order to have optimum health, you should only eat grass fed animals. You should only be eating organic fruits and vegetables. Food that is grown organically has the most viable energy structure, and it promotes our lives. We feel younger, we do not get diseased, and the food passes more naturally through our system. We no longer get fat, and our vitality is increased.

Your diet should be completely organic; however, this can be expensive. You should do your best to live closely to these guidelines as possible, however. Eat fruits, vegetables, and drink lots of water. If you like to eat meat, go for it. You should start taking steps toward a healthier lifestyle. You must be willing to make adjustments here and there.

Much of the food you already eat is essentially cardboard. Poisons, lack of proper feeding, and horrible chemicals have stripped basically all of the nutrients away from many of our fruits, vegetables, and meats. At the end of the day, we are left to be even more bloated, acidic, and toxic.

It may cost a little more, or even a lot more, but you must make this switch. Your life really depends on it. Sugary, processed, goods only make life worse for you. It's time to really make changes in our lives.

Instead of spending money on beer, candies, cigarettes, and other foolish expenditures, throw some money towards health. It's funny how when someone wants something badly enough, he or she will ALWAYS find away. Usually, the desire is something like making enough money, buying a house, getting married, buying a video game, going to a sporting event, a concert, etc.; however, when it comes to health, peoples' wallets tighten.

Take care of yourself, take care of your body, take care of your soul! Everything else will take care of itself. Your action today is to go to your kitchen and take account of all the food you have. Take out anything that does not serve you. Take inventory the cookies, the candies, the sodas, the beers, the chocolates, the white breads, the jams, the ice creams, and anything else that does not serve you. If you can, throw them away. If not, feel free to keep them until they finish. It would be best to throw that stuff out, though.

Next, go online and try to find organic variations of them. As one product finishes, buy its organic variation from henceforth. Try buying all your fruits and vegetables organically as well. They don't taste any different, but they will end up making you feel millions of times better in the long run. It's not what we do once in a while that impacts our health, it's what we do consistently. Feel free to reward yourself with an unhealthy snack from time to time. This way, you will not feel imprisoned by a new lifestyle. Flexibility is everything. As long as organic eating is your habit, it's okay to sneak in devils of junk sparingly.

Conclusion

You have made it the beginning of your journey- yes, I said beginning. You have a new life now, and you must constantly nurture it. The practices lain in this book will take you to unbelievable levels of health, love, and joy. You must take all of these practices into consideration, and you must apply them with all of your heart. You must believe that you are already healed. You must have faith without needing proof, because believing is seeing. You must never give up the fight. We must work together to make this world a place filled with love and health. Every single dream you could have ever imagined can come true, but you must let it happen. Have faith, and know that if you desire it, it **must** come to pass.

You are now a dissenter. I have shown you the way out of the Cave. It is now your job to bring more people into the sunlight. When we take our lives into our own hands, it empowers us. We must look at the world and realize we are creating every moment which we are a part of. I have taught you that belief is everything. Hopefully you went through this training regiment as prescribed. If you have just read through this book in order to get the gist, great! Now, you must go back and actually follow the routine.

If you believe in yourself, if you believe that you already have the very thing that you desire, if you spread love to the world, if you focus on the very thing that you want, you will vibrate your wishes into existence. No pill can replace the power of the human mind and a pursuit backed by faith.

God Bless
Chet Anthony Johnson

Works Cited

Braden, Gregg. *Fractal Time: the Secret of 2012 and a New World Age*. Carlsbad, Calif.: Hay House, 2010. Print.

"A Brief History of Time - Stephen W. Hawking." *Generation Terrorists*. Web. 22 June 2010. <http://www.generationterrorists.com/quotes/abhotswh.html>.

Bruce, Robert. *Astral Dynamics: the Complete Book of Out-of-body Experiences*. Charlottesville, VA: Hampton Roads Pub., 2009. Print.

By. "What Happens When We Die? - TIME." *Breaking News, Analysis, Politics, Blogs, News Photos, Video, Tech Reviews - TIME.com*. Web. 21 June 2010. <http://www.time.com/time/health/article/0,8599,1842627,00.html>.

"Detailed Listing of Acid / Alkaline Forming Foods." *Jeff Rense Program*. Web. 21 June 2010. <http://www.rense.com/1.mpicons/acidalka.htm>.

Hawkins, David R. *Power vs. Force: the Hidden Determinants of Human Behavior*. Carlsbad, Calif.: Hay House, 2002. Print.

"Holonomic Brain Theory - Scholarpedia." *Main Page - Scholarpedia*. Web. 21 June 2010. <http://www.scholarpedia.org/article/Holonomic_brain_theory>.

"How the Marx Brothers Brought Norman Cousins Back to Life." *The Healing Power of Laughter*. Web. 22 June 2010. <http://thehealingpoweroflaughter.blogspot.com/2007/07/how-marx-brothers-brought-norman.html>.

"IAVH - History of Homoeopathy." *IAVH - International Association for Veterinary Homoeopathy*. Web. 22 June 2010. <http://www.iavh.org/homeopathy/history/>.

"Lesson 18 - Restoring PH Balance in the Body." *Natural Health School*. Web. 22 June 2010.
   <http://www.naturalhealthschool.com/pH-balance.html>.

Long, Jeffrey, and Paul Perry. *Evidence of the Afterlife: the Science of Near-death Experiences*. New York: HarperOne, 2010. Print.

"Products." *Christopher Howard Trainingâ,, ¢*. Web. 21 June 2010.
   <http://www.chrishoward.com/Public/ProductDescriptions/index.cfm>.